DETOX OR DIEt

Closing the Gap between Dis-Ease and Death

ALSO BY KELLEY (Kelly) R. PORTER

Perfectly Planned (Overcoming Incest, Rape & Sexual Abuse)

Perfectly Planned Workbook and Audiobook

Overcoming Toxic Relationships (Creating Power from Past Pain)

Mental MakeOver (Creating a Positive Mindset) Book of Quotes

It's All About Life (Book of Poems)

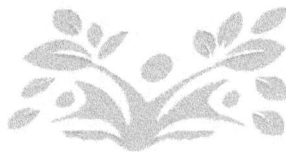

COACH KELLEY
TRANSFORMING LIVES WORLDWIDE

DETOX OR DIEt

Closing the Gap between Dis-Ease and Death

KELLEY R PORTER, MLT, ASCP, LIFE COACH

WITH CONTRIBUTIONS FROM RICHARD ALEXANDER, M.D., N.D., JENN STAGG, N.D., & JANET HULL STARR, PH.D.

Designed by Kelley Porter
Cover Created by Kelley Porter
Library of Congress Control Number:
ISBN: 978-0-9851767-6-1

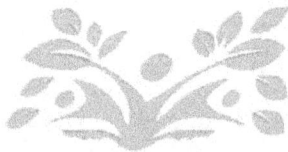

PORTER PUBLISHING
TRANSFORMING LIVES WORLDWIDE

Nothing contained in this book is intended to establish a physician-patient relationship, to replace the services of a trained physician or health care professional, or otherwise to be a substitute for professional medical advice, diagnosis, or treatment. Information in this book is a combination of information found via research, medical literature and through my direct experience as well as working with medical doctors, naturopaths, holistic practitioners and plant practitioners. Nothing, including communications with Kelley Porter should be taken as medical advice. Because of the risk involved, the author of this book is not responsible for any opposing detoxification effects or consequences resulting from the use of any suggestions or procedures described in this book. Please check with your doctor or nutritionist before making any dietary changes or starting any cleansing or detox programs. The author and publisher of this book have used their best efforts in preparing this document. The author and publisher make no representation or warranties with respect to the accuracy, applicability or completeness of the contents of this document. The information contained in this document is for educational purposes. Therefore, if you wish to apply ideas contained in this book, you are completely accountable for your actions. The author and publisher shall in no way be held liable to any party for any direct, indirect, punitive, special, incidental or other consequential damages that may arise from direct or indirect use of this material. The material in this book is provided "as is" and without warranties. As always, the advice of a skilled doctor or other health professional should be sought. All links are for information purposes only and are not warranted for content, accuracy or any other implied or explicit purpose.

With love, honor and gratitude
This book is dedicated to my husband,
Patrick O. Turner,
and our son,
Shemar Cooper,
who have tremendously supported me
throughout my healing journey,
I love them so.

It is imperative for this book that I share my love, and gratitude to those who have supported, educated and assisted me in creating this work of art. Rita Stewart, an author, and CEO of Master Force Inc., a private organization that offers one of the most robust coaching certification programs. I thank you, Rita, for creating a program that has completely transformed my being as well as elevated my business. The wealth and abundance I create in my life today are because of Master Force. Thank you for being a phenomenal woman.

Marc Haygood, a certified nutritionist, plant practitioner and author, taught me what it means to be a health and wellness coach advocate. I thank Marc Haygood for his detox program as without his presence and meeting him when I did; I can assure you I would not be writing this book. I also thank Marc for continuously assisting me along my health and wellness journey.

Richard Anderson, (Founder of Arise & Shine) is a naturopathic doctor, medical researcher, nutritionist, iridologist, and herbalist. I have much gratitude for Dr. Anderson for trusting me with his work as I have never physically met him, but only via email. Dr. Anderson graciously contributed his expertise on mucoid plaque and allowed me to add a section from his new book (Transformational Cleanse) to the book you're reading now.

Jenn Stagg, N.D., and author of Unzip Your Genes and owner of the integrative specialty practice, Whole Health Wellness Center. Dr. Stagg is a well-known expert in integrative medicine and has appeared on NBC, CBS and ABC. I am grateful for Dr. Stagg's permission to utilize her article on thoughts, emotions, and disease. I have never met her but chatted with her via email.

Jack Zoldan, a board-certified Internal Medicine physician that combines traditional and alternative nutritional and lifestyle therapies to help people improve their health by taking control of their own lives. I am grateful Dr. Zoldan took time from his busy schedule to talk to me about a documentary project as he permitted me to use information from his website on Candida yeast.

Janet Starr Hull, PH.D, author, nutritionist, and toxicologist contributed to Detox or Diet by permitting the use of her article on parasites destroyers. In 1991, Dr. Hull had an unexpected change in career after her Grave's disease diagnosis. Through diligent research and her thorough understanding of toxicity, she later discovered her "Grave's Disease" was aspartame poisoning. She has since worked to inform consumers about the health dangers of artificial sweeteners.

Regina Thomas Dillard, author, and Raw, Living Food Chef introduced me to my first raw, live and vegan lasagna. I thank Regina for allowing me to include her delicious recipe in my book. Please find Regina's recipe book "Feed" in stores today.

Being taught to do better doesn't mean you have applied the tools to do better. People that know better actually do better.
-CoachKelley

Contents

Holistic Health, Medicine, Money & Parasites 1
Emotional Toxins.. 11
Burning From the Inside 27
Self-Diagnosis 42
Lichen Planus Diagnosis 57
Light Therapy 68
Turpentine and Castor Oil 78
Detox and Colon Cleanse 92
Worms, Worms, Worms 114
Healing Crisis Symptoms 124
Eat To Live 145
Illness Raises Your Vibrations...................................... 165
Pain Creates Power and Purpose 180
Gratitude 185
Natural Healing Remedies (Dr. Hull) 187
Conclusion 194

Epilogue
Questions
References
About the Author

I easily flow with change. My life is Divinely guided and I am always going in the right direction.

- Louis Hay

Do you feel tired, fatigued, can't remember anything or lose words in the middle of a sentence? Do you feel like something is crawling on you, but you can't find the bug? Do you have digestive problems like irritable bowel syndrome, colitis, inflammatory bowel disease, flatulence (gas) that won't quit, or bloating? Do you suffer from food sensitivities or food allergies? How many allergic reactions have you experienced and doctors couldn't tell you why? Do you have severe cravings for sugar? Have you experienced persistent vaginal yeast infections and have no idea why? How many times have your doctor told you he or she has no idea where the disease comes from or the cause is unknown? Do your joints hurt? Did you lose weight and gain it back even while exercising on a regular? Do you have trouble losing weight? Well, everything mentioned above was me as recently I discovered I was a walking human host for several different worms and an overgrowth of candida yeast. Over the years, I experienced more dis-ease than I can imagine and the sad part is most of them always came back after I took a prescribed pill from the doctor. And so that we are clear, here is a list of every symptom (dis-ease), I have ever experienced in my 46 years of life and no particular order.

- Inflammatory Bowel Disease
- Colitis (inflammation of the colon)
- Irritable Bowel Syndrome (IBS)
- Floaters and flashes in my eyes
- Chills, fever
- Inability to sweat
- Unspecified sweating
- Hot flashes
- Psoriasis, Pityriasis Rosea, acne
- Lichen Planus

- Yeast infections
- Insomnia
- Anxiety
- Teeth grinding: (Bruxemia)
- Anal itch
- Chronic fatigue
- Allergies
- Sinus pressure
- Pneumonia
- Alopecia
- Depression
- Influenza
- Bronchitis
- Common cold
- Constipation, diarrhea, bloating and gas
- Joint and muscle pain
- Dark circles around or under the eyes
- Brain fog or poor coordination
- Early stage heart disease
- Hypothyroidism
- Obesity
- High Blood Pressure
- High Cholesterol

I am sure I am missing something, but you get the point. In all that illness, there is one thing for sure that has helped me tremendously, and that has been diet and nutrition. However, you might wonder why certain dis-ease returns. Well, if you don't rid your body of the source, the dis-ease will return. That source is parasites. After currently releasing several different worms, and candida yeast from my body, I am one hundred percent convinced they are the root of all the symptoms or dis-ease mentioned and your doctors might have no idea at all. After you finish this book, share it with your family, friends, school, doctors, neighbors, church, neighborhood clinic, health market and anyone else who you believe might benefit. We were trained to rely on doctors to heal us. But, how can doctors cure us if they have no idea that parasitic infections in the United States exist and are rapidly increasing? Doctors are trained to believe parasitic diseases occur more in foreign or third world countries. How can they help us if their ignorance runs deeper than the rabbit hole? How can they help us if they believe they are diagnosing proper dis-ease?

The healthcare industry is no different than logistics, information technology, theology, politics, economics and any other field of study. These areas of research grant you a job and create a paycheck for you. Nowhere in the history of earth has medicine ever healed the real source of disease. Holistic or homeopathic healing and nutrition was the original method and the only actual sources of treating the body. However, we must get to the root of the health crisis in America, and that is parasites or yeast and worms. As you continue to read, triggers will occur, unstable emotions will arise, as will disbelief. And that is okay. I just encourage you to open your mind to unlearn, learn and relearn. The healthcare industry is a trillion dollar industry. The healthcare insurance companies and the pharmaceutical companies are billion dollar industries. The food industry is a trillion dollar industry. And how do you think they profit? These corporations benefit from us, the sick and dis-eased Americans.

The best weapon we can have is education and truth as I hope that Detox or DIEt will become a beacon of light for every individual in our world.

Health and Wellness
15% Exercise
85% what you eat
100% what you think
1000% how you feel

Kelley Porter

CHAPTER ONE

Holistic Health, Medicine, Money and Parasites

Make no mistake about it, worms are the most toxic agents in the human body. They are one of the primary underlying causes of disease and are the most basic cause of a compromised immune system.
Hazel Parcells, D.C., N.D., Ph.D., 1974

I strongly believe that every patient with disorder of immune function, including multiple allergies (especially food allergies), and patients with unexplained fatigue or chronic bowel symptoms should be evaluated for the presence of intestinal parasites.
Leo Galland, M.D.
Townsend Letter for Doctors, 1988

We have a tremendous parasite problem right here in the United States – it's just not being identified.
Peter Weina, Ph.D., Chief of Pathobiology,
Walter Reed Army Institute of Research, 1991

Instead of healing people, the broken healthcare system is prolonging people's suffering in too many cases. Instead of preventing epidemics, it is generating them.
John E. Sarno. M.D., 2007

I released hundreds of worms from my body (pinworms, roundworms, tapeworms and liver flukes.) Some were very long and some were about an inch long. The smell reeked of sewage.
Kelley Porter, MLT, ASCP, Certified Life Coach, 2017

In the 1700's, treatment for the ill consisted of herbs such as senna, aloe, figs and castor oil (Mullins, 1988). Senna leaf is a natural anti-parasitic herb that relieves constipation and expels parasites from the body. Aspidium roots (the male fern), pomegranate bark, and wormseed oil treated intestinal (Mullins, 1988). Even in this modern day, herbalist and holistic healers currently use castor oil, aloe vera juice or the plant, as well as turpentine. And wouldn't you know it, aloe vera destroys parasites as well. I used several of them to expel the parasites that hijacked my body. One of the doctors I visited at the University of Chicago hospital told me to stop doing herbal enemas as senna causes the colon to darken or melanosis. I found that to be interesting as I had not used senna or any product containing senna.

In the east, santonin flowers healed parasitic infections as it also is an anti-parasitic that rids the body of parasites (Mullins, 1988). In the Western half of the globe, holistic doctors used chenopodium, a plant that kills parasites (online dictionary).

You're probably wondering where I am going with this information. Well, why was healing based on killing and expelling parasites from the body? Why was every herb used considered an anti-parasitic plant or herb? Why? All the flowers used for healing exterminated parasitic diseases. Otherwise, why focus on plants that killed parasites? Removing the worms initiated healing. As you continue to read, you will understand how holistic health in America became about how to make money not healing.

Pain relievers were alcohol, hyoscyamus leaves, and opium. Hyoscyamus containing scopolamine was used to actuate "twilight sleep" in modern medicine. Hyoscyamus was recommended to alleviate over-excitability, restlessness, and general disruptive behavior in hyperactive children (Unknown author). In the sixteenth century, Arabs utilized colchicum, a saffron derivative, for rheumatic pains and gout (Mullins, 1988). Snap bark, the source of quinine, treated malaria; chaulmoogra oil treated leprosy, and ipecac treated amoebic dysentery (Mullins, 1988). There is it again, ipecac and quinine; treats parasites

2

(malaria and amoebic dysentery). However, there was more holistic healing such as burned sponge and its content iodine, managed and cured goiters and midwives utilized ergot to contract the uterus (Mullins, 1988).

Until the late nineteenth century, doctors practiced as independent agents, which meant that they assumed all of the risks for any medical error. The poor didn't have access to doctors as medical cures were only for the rich and powerful. To balance out the potential risk of these free-lance doctors, Mullins (1988) believed that was the beginning of the medical monopoly. Some two hundred years ago, the era of modern medicine was ushered in by Sir Humphry Davy's discovery of the anesthetic properties of nitrous oxide (Mullins, 1988).

As you can see, holistic or natural healing are not secrets to the healthcare industry, however, when you have people like Rockefeller controlling and implementing new ways to monopolize, the healthcare industry becomes about the bottom line and not healing. What's more, leaving the poor to die is just as common today in modern medicine. The attempts to build up this medical monopoly have now created a modern plague, costing the public dearly in money and suffering (Mullins, 1988).

Almost five centuries ago, one of the first attempts to set up this monopoly took place in England. The Act of 1511, signed into law by King Henry the 8th, in England, made it an offense to practice physic or surgery without the approval of a panel of "experts" (Mullins, 1988). That brings me to Dr. Sebi and how he was arrested and spent two years in prison for "practicing" medicine. While in court, the judge asked him was he practicing medicine, and he responded, your doctors are practicing medicine, I'm healing people; priceless. However, Dr. Sebi spent two years in prison for treating people and violating the dictator's laws of practicing medicine. Dr. Sebi did not have any medical degrees, yet he cured Aids, impotence, diabetes and other disease using natural herbs.

Formed in 1518 along with the founding of the Royal College of Physicians, this act granted the same powers to barbers and surgeons in 1540 when the King approved their companies (Mullins, 1988). A campaign to eliminate unauthorized practitioners who served the poor was immediately launched (Mullins, 1988). That hasn't changed today. How many stories have you heard of uninsured people not receiving medical care as they could not pay for services? The Emergency Medical Treatment and Active Labor Act (EMTALA), also known as the "Patient Anti-Dumping," prohibited emergency rooms from refusing treatment to those who were uninsured or could not afford to pay. Hospital emergency rooms rejected many poor people and were sued by some. Unfortunately, that tragedy still occurs today so the Emtala law doesn't hold much substance.

This harassment of doctors who served the poor caused such widespread suffering in England that King Henry the 8th was forced to enact the Quacks Charter in 1542. This Charter exempted the "unauthorized practitioners" and allowed them to continue their treatments, (Mullins, 1988). In America, that law doesn't exist as you can see Dr. Sebi spent two years in jail for "practicing" medicine as he does not hold an M.D. and is not a member of the American Medical Association (AMA). However, in past times, Dr. Sebi would be considered a quack. Medical disclaimers are very important to those who provide holistic healing and do not have a doctor of medicine.

Shameful, however, because, holistic healing works as you will understand once you delve into my story. During the entire year of my healing crisis, I used 5 milligrams of steroids for five days and four pills to kill the worms. After that, everything I used came from the ground.

In 1832, the British Medical Association became the drive for the forming of the American Association in the United States. From inception, the AMA has had one principal objective, and that was to attain and defend a monopoly of the practice of medicine in the United States (Mullins, 1988). From its creation, the AMA

4

made allopathy the basis of its tradition (Mullins, 1988). Allopathy was a type of medicine whose practitioners had received training in a recognized academic school of medicine and relied heavily on surgical procedures and the use of medications (Mullins, 1988). In Germany, the initiators of this form of healing frequently used bleeding techniques and large doses of drugs (Mullins, 1988). What's more, the Germans were unfriendly to anyone who did not follow the allopathy procedures (Mullins, 1988). So, there you have it. Modern medicine has four principles, and they are money, bleeding, surgery, and drugs. Nowhere in their empire does it state anything about healing or creating better health. In fact, even to this day, M.D's are so indoctrinated that they believe their methods work.

In 1854, a breakout of Cholera resulted in 16.4% deaths in homeopathic hospitals and 50% deaths in traditional or conventional medical hospitals (Mullins, 1988). That record was silenced and covered up by the Board of Health of the City of London. What's more, clinical trials have proved that homeopathy is just as effective as arthritic drugs if not better and that they produced no side effects (Mullins, 1988). Homeopathic healing has no side effects, but let's look at some of the side effects pharmaceutical drugs cause. Pharmaceutical drugs cause dizziness, dry mouth, headache; sleep problems (insomnia); feeling nervous or irritable; fever, hot flashes, sweating; pounding heartbeats or fluttering in your chest; changes in your menstrual periods; or appetite changes, weight changes. Those were the side effects from taking Levothyroxine for hypothyroidism. Why would anyone be convinced to take drugs and not know how to detox their body? If doctors are required to write prescriptions, then they should be required to teach patients how to detox their bodies. But that would necessitate a course on nutrition, herbs, and supplements leading to a healed body and exterminate the pharmaceutical companies and doctors.

Traditional or conventional medicine is about bleeding, removing body parts, drugs and money. Conventional medicine has and never will surround healing. As you read more, you witness that I healed my body without doctors and drugs. In fact, the University of Chicago hospital doctors did absolutely nothing to improve my skin or treat the real problems. As long as you and I have good insurance, we will receive a pill and a bill. The American healthcare system is a complete scam and created on the idea of making money.

In 1892, Rockefeller appointed Frederick T. Gates as the head of all his humanitarian endeavors. As it turned out, each of Rockefeller's efforts was explicitly created to increase not only his wealth and power but also the wealth and power of those he represented (Mullins, 1988). Frederick T. Gates' first present to Rockefeller was a plan to dominate the entire medical education system in the United States. Rockefeller organization initiated the first steps, and his education board spent more than $100 million to gain control of the nation's medical schools and turn our physicians to physicians of the allopathic school (Mullins, 1988). Again, allopathically refers to the mainstream medical use of pharmaceutical drugs, and physical interventions to treat or suppress symptoms or pathophysiologic processes of diseases or conditions. In lay terms, suppress your immune system as it is your immune system that responds to any crises in the body such as dis-ease and provokes symptoms of the disease. So, how does mainstream medicine heal anyone? It doesn't and never will. Mainstream medicine has cured cancer, sexually transmitted diseases, bronchitis, and other dis-eases, but, at the expense of creating more illness or dis-ease in your body. What's more, the real creator of disease is toxins. Toxins like, worms, yeast, GMO's, emotional and thought-form toxins, mucoid plaque, street drugs, pharmaceutical drugs and much more. But again, drugs don't heal; they kill but while in medical school, doctors are taught drugs heal.

The medical education system was so elitist, expensive and very drawn out that most students couldn't consider a medical career (Mullins, 1988). The Flexner program set up requirements for four years of undergraduate college, and a further four years of medical school. His report also set up complex requirements for the medical schools; they must have expensive laboratories and other equipment (Mullins, 1988). Before the Rockefeller medical monopoly, America was the most significant and productive nation in the world because we had the healthiest citizens in the world. In 1910, when Rockefeller organization took over the medical profession our citizens went into a sharp decline (Mullins, 1988). Today, we suffer from a host of debilitating ailments, both mental and physical, nearly all of which can be traced directly to the operations of the chemical and drug monopoly, and which pose the most significant threat to our continued existence as a nation (Mullins, 1988). If you don't learn anything from this chapter or book, I need you to learn how to take control of your health.

To take control of your health, you must understand why you are sick. According to Gittleman (1993), parasites are an insidious public health threat in the United States today. Insidious because so very few people are talking about parasites, and even fewer people are listening (Gittleman 1993). My question is why? Why do people not want to hear about parasites and what could be the real reason we are sick. If knowing the truth helped me live a long and healthy life, then I want the facts and regardless of how gross it is. You understand that doctors are clueless about parasitic infections, so who else is going to teach you? How will you know what's deteriorating your health if your only options are doctors and medicine? How many times have you heard someone say parasite infections are in third world countries? How many times have you heard someone say parasite infections associate with poor hygiene and malnutrition? I've heard it a lot and even in school when I studied parasitology. The education surrounding parasites was that they were more common in places like Africa, and Asia. So many lies taught by the Rockefeller Corporation. What's more, physicians do not suspect or recognize the symptoms of a parasitic infection. As a medical laboratory technician, parasitology and microbiology were two areas I studied. I have witnessed and reported one case of malaria in America. What's more, I have seen and diagnosed yeast candida in the blood of patients as well as parasites after testing for ova

7

and parasites. Parasitic infections in American are just as prevalent as diabetes, and they may just be related. Parasitic infection not only affects the digestive system, but the endocrine system as well.

In the United States, physicians are not educated in parasitology and therefore very inexperienced in recognizing typical clinical symptoms. You will witness that as I discuss my experience with doctors at the University of Chicago hospital. If they have any education on parasitology, it may be a minor or an introduction via a microbiology chapter (Gittleman 1993). Parasitology is an area of specialty within the infectious disease department. However, if doctors think parasite related disorders are limited to third world countries, why would they ever suspect Americans are suffering from parasitic infections? If you don't question it, they will never treat it. In 1976 the Center for Disease Control revealed that one in every six people had one or more parasites (Gittleman 1993). That was three decades ago. Imagine how many people are infected with parasites today. Well, according to the World Health Organization, 3.5 billion people suffer from some type of parasitic infection. Based on Gittleman's experience, projections for the year 2025 suggest that more than half of the 8 billion people on earth will be infected.

According to Gittleman (1993), warning signs of parasitic infections are constipation, diarrhea, gas and bloating, irritable bowel syndrome, joint and muscle pain, anemia, allergies, skin conditions, granulomas, chronic fatigue and immune dysfunction. Does any of that sound familiar? Keep reading as you will witness that I have had a parasitic infection for over three decades and more than likely, you have too.

Based on my education and previous position as Medical Lab Technologist, there are several tests used to diagnose parasite infections. The first one is ova (egg) and parasite (worm) test (o&p). This analysis is performed on the stool and used to find parasites that cause diarrhea, cramping, gas and other abdominal illness. The center for disease control (cdc) recommends that three or more stool samples, collected on separate days, be examined. A colonoscopy is also used to find parasites that cause diarrhea, cramping, flatulence and other abdominal symptoms. However, the colonoscopy does not examine the small intestine. Therefore worms can be missed. Blood tests such as serology and a blood smear that look for antibodies or parasite antigens when the body's immune system fights off infections. The blood smear is also examined via the use of a microscope and looks for parasites such as malaria or babesiosis. A complete blood draw (cbc) is also performed to test for increased eosinophils as high eosinophil counts represent parasitic infection among other conditions.

Lastly, Magnetic Resonance Imaging (MRI) and Computerized Axial Tomography scan (CAT). These tests are used to look for some parasitic diseases that may cause lesions in the organs. Doctors probably diagnose those same wounds as cancer. I might be wrong, but how would you know? Has any doctor ever told you where any cancer originated? No, and they never will as they have no idea. All disease starts with toxins. We don't catch cancer; toxins in the body create it.

How would you know if parasites aren't the underlying cause of your failing health? We are all responsible for our health as doctors are not responsible for us. So, take your power back. Doctors neglect the fact that parasites might be the underlying reason for all of your dis-ease as the symptoms mimic a host of other ailments. According to Gittelman (1993), pinworms are at the seat of your child's hyperactivity, irritable bowel syndrome and giardia may cause chronic fatigue. Roundworm infection may cause persistent allergies (Gittelman 1993).

However, don't be fooled, emotions (spiritually speaking) are the start of all mind-body disorder. When the body finally manifests dis-ease, you better believe there is a corresponding toxic emotion. But let us not forget that there is a spiritual or emotional element of dis-ease. According to Hay (1999), the presence of parasites means giving power to others, letting them

9

take over. More than half of Americans are guilty of relinquishing their control over to the education system, the religious and healthcare system.

So, what do we do, we take our power back. How do we take our power back? We empower ourselves with real education and the truth. We recognize that all disease starts in mind first and then manifest itself as mind-body disorder. We learn how to love and accept ourselves. We arm ourselves with "real" food and eat to live and not live it eat. We learn how to detox our elimination channels and cleanse our colon. We understand that we are Gods and Goddesses and the power is within us, not in a church or the pastor. We know that best education is "experiences" and not the American educational system. And if you haven't had the experiences then learn from someone who has. Take your power back and take control of your health and wellness.

CHAPTER TWO

Emotional Toxins

Driving east on 127th street towards I-94 as I approached the end of the road, I quickly swerved over to the left and panicky back to the right lane. A dead dear lied in the middle of the road, and as I swerved to the left, I almost hit a car head on. My heart beat fast as I was scared shitless. *What is to come of this day? Damn, I could've died.* I thought. I continued driving and jumped onto I-94 and drove to Hammond Indiana to punch the clock for a laboratory. I had no idea what events would occur this particular day, but that dead deer symbolized something. I felt heavy, sad and like my soul had died. On that day, the conflict within me was loud, and I had to make a decision. I walked back and forth at my workstation trying to hold my tears back. I talked to one of my co-workers and the lead tech. Eventually, I shared my truth with the supervisor and the manager. Before talking to my supervisors, I called my husband.

"Hello."
"Hey, Pat."
"What's wrong?" Pat could hear the agony in my trembling voice.
"I can't do this anymore."
"Do what? Work, punch the clock, I feel like I'm dying in here. I want to quit."
"When?"
"Right now."
"Are you serious?"
"Yes."
"So, you're going to quit doing what you love and never look back."
"Yes, Pat I believe in myself and I need you to believe in me. I need your support. If you decide you don't want to support me, we can get a divorce."
"I don't need to hear all that. Are you sure that's what you want to do?"

"Yes, I'm sure."

"Okay, then quit."

"I can quit."

"If that's what you want and to pursue your dreams, then go ahead."

"Thank you, Pat." I cried. Joy filled my heart at that moment.

"I have to tell the boss now."

"Okay, I will see you when you get home."

That was all I needed. The support of my husband lit a fire under my ass, and the rest is history. For so long, I didn't believe I could work for myself, make a living and do great at it. I always thought I needed a job. I felt it was the only way to survive. I was wrong. In fact, I never thought I was good enough to have my own business. But, something came over me that day, and that was the day I took that jump that Steve Harvey discussed. I shared the news with the supervisors, and they were not happy at all. In fact, the boss told me, *I would like to see you make it without a job.* I was shocked he said that, but what could I expect from someone who believed that was the only way to live. I walked out that door and never looked back.

I remember walking in about a 4 inches of snow to my car and thinking everything was going to be okay. I sat in my car filled with mixed emotions. I sat there thinking, what next. I tapped camera on my Samsung S6, placed my phone on the inside of my steering wheel and poured my heart out.

Good Morning,

Coach Kelley here feeling a little inspired, empowered, and courageous. I started an assignment almost three months ago at this laboratory in Indiana. And the whole time I've been here these three months; I felt like my soul was burning every time I came in here. You know, I was off work for a year and a half and that year and a half did justice for my business. Am I a millionaire? No, but do I have the talent and potential and the gifs to live the life I deserve? Yes, I do. And I might get emotional because I literally just walked out this damn place, not because they did anything, but because I ain't happy there, I don't wanna be there. And of course, the bosses wanna try to talk me into it ... and tell me if you abandon your job, you know...it's going to be a mark on your work history. I don't care. What I do care about is my happiness and I have faith in the Universe that this jump that I just took is going to pan out just fine.

I'm sharing this to you guys because don't stay anywhere you are not happy. Don't. Because it just brings more unhappiness to your soul, to your person, your family, everything, (crying). I never thought I would just walk without like a resignation letter or anything like that, but at this point in time I have too many talents and gifts to be working for any damn body and if I have to struggle my ass off getting where I want to get, I'm going to do it (crying).

But I ain't punching no more clocks. I'm not punching anymore clocks. This shit takes too much time away from me writing books, coaching clients and you know... just doing the things I truly have desire for and passion for. So again, if you ain't happy where you at, just leave and have faith that the Universe will provide, believe in yourself, and trust the process of life and everything will be okay. (Crying, today is what, February 2nd, 3rd, I don't know what it is, but this is a new journey for me. I ain't punching no more damn clocks and Imma be just fine. Like this message, share this message, 'cus somebody needs to hear it. Don't worry about materialistic things that you may or may not be able to get.

Peace and sanity is the most important thing in my life and I had a dose of that the year and a half I was off and I ain't giving it back to nobody. I'm not giving it back to nobody. Imma take my ass home, finish my sixth book, Imma keep writing, keep empowering and Imma keep changing lives. Imma keep doing exactly what it is I want to do. I'm sorry I had to walk away the way I did, but shit, you know, these jobs don't care about us. All they care about is a body and their money, they don't care about us. They don't care about the talents and gifts that God has blessed us with. They don't care about that. All they see is you as a body and you working them eight hours; slaving you. I am not doing it anymore. I'm about to put my damn seatbelt (leaning forward) on and go home where my husband supports and is waiting for me and Imma continue to change some lives (while fixing my wig). In the meantime, y'all have a wonderful day (chuckles) and I love y'all. Bye.

Video link
https://www.facebook.com/KelleyPorterT/videos/2250542244 97037/

The last time I checked (September 2017), over 25,000 people viewed that video. February 2nd was the day my life completely changed and all for the better, but as you read, you might think differently.

Metaphysically or spiritually speaking, the dead dear meant conflict. That conflict was in me and bigger than I imagined. I knew it was time for me to stop punching the clock, believe in myself and live on purpose. But, I was afraid to believe beyond what I knew I was capable of. On that day, February 2, 2016, I stepped out on faith and took that jump that Steve Harvey spoke of as there have been many speed bumps and potholes in the road. I am so grateful for my husband's support, however, what came six months later, drastically changed my entire life. The conflict was more profound than taking a "jump" as I learned just how deep it was.

As time moved on, I realized how unsatisfied I was without the money I used to have as I wasn't able to care for my son the way I used to and help my husband. I felt worthless as I hated myself. I was utterly miserable on the inside, and those unhealthy emotions trickled down into my marriage. What I didn't realize was those same emotions were manifesting a sickness in me that I didn't know lived inside me. I was angry and hated myself for the decision I made. I felt broke within my entire being. I harbored those unhealthy emotions for almost two months and projected my pain onto Patrick.

Many days I set at my computer for twelve hours creating products that would not only help the Universe but generate income. I didn't give Pat much attention as I thought working was what he wanted me to do. I recalled from the previous year he was kind enough to let me quit working (the first time) and follow my purpose, but he also wanted me to go back to work after a year.

A part of me did as well, at that time as I still didn't entirely believe in myself. However, I sat, day in and out at my computer feeling like shit on the inside. Even with clients, I didn't feel like I was doing enough and not because of Pat, but because I connected my worth with money, how much I had, how much I could do and how much I could spend. That was the worst thing I could've ever done.

Everything I felt took not only away from me, but my marriage. My emotions were scattered and unhealthy as they carried a lot of weight, but mentally and physically. Emotions are energy in motion and as we all know energy is transferable. I know Patrick and Shemar felt the weight of my pain. It was heavy and as I stated before, a lot more than I thought. I cried many days when I was alone. Too many days my son wanted, and I could not provide. Shemar never went without his needs met, but I desired to fill his wants as I have always done. Pat's income wasn't enough to sustain the lifestyle I conditioned myself to live, and I certainly didn't want to make him responsible for the upkeep of the life I created for my son.

Although, I knew all I had to do was ask and Patrick would've worked fifty hours a week to give me whatever I desired. But, my pride wouldn't allow me to ask as my son's wants wasn't as crucial as his needs. At any rate, I went on suffering in silence. I didn't know how to live without a job. My father just told me to go to college and get a good job, and I did that. No one ever told me I could have my own business, live happily and stable without a job. I almost attached to my boss's words. His words were embedded in my subconscious mind as I completely believed I could not make it in life without a job. At this time, you might wonder, what that has to do with my health.

Emotional and mental health quadrants are two aspects of the life quadrant and if my emotional and psychological health is scattered and unstable, what exactly do you think will happen to my physical health?

If one is to have optimal health, one has to balance their overall being, and that includes your mindset, emotions, physical body, and spirituality. Three months passed and "stinking thinking" and destructive emotions filled my heart and mind.

I recall one night in March as I couldn't sleep; Pat had just come home from work as I wrote in another book. Around one o'clock in the morning, I awoke him.

"Pat, will you please wake up? I need to talk to you as I cried with my head hung low."

"Hey, hey, what's wrong? Pat arose out of bed and sat next to me."

Crying, "I just don't know what to do. I'm trying, and I'm working as much as I can. I sit at that computer sometimes twelve hours a day creating products and programs. I feel worthless as I can't help you or provide the things that Shemar wants. I don't know how to live without a job. I feel worthless."

"Wow. Baby it's going to be okay." Pat wiped his eyes. "I feel worthless sometimes to as I want you and Shemar to have everything you need and want and I feel worthless that I'm not able to give it to you both."

"Are you serious?" I wiped my eyes and felt a sense of relief and not only from my release, but Pat understood me and felt the same way. That moment freed me from those toxic emotions. "Baby, so what do we do?"

"You continue to believe in yourself, and we will be just fine. If I have to work a few extra hours, then so be it."

"Thank you. I love you." I said as I cried. I also wanted to say; I'm sorry for withholding sex and neglecting you. My emotions were everywhere, as I felt so detached and not from you, but from myself."

"You're welcome baby." We 'gon be just fine. You are right where you are supposed to be; at home doing what you do and helping people heal. Hell, you're helping me too."

"Thank you. I feel so much better now. I wish I had said something sooner to you. I just thought you wanted me to work hard."

"I thought you wanted me to work fifty hours a week."

"Nope. I prefer you just work the hours your boss assigned you and come home. I don't want you to enslave yourself for those people. You have a family, and we need you at home as well and not always tired."

"Wow. Damn. Thank you. I needed to hear that. That's good to know." We both laughed. "Okay, well good. Now that we got that out the way come here and make love to me."

That ten-minute dialogue set my mind free as I was able to release those toxic emotions. I was able to make love to my husband and move forward in my life and purpose. I felt good after that day, but as we know life, there is always something that will show up to teach us even more. I was grateful not to have to go back to punching the clock as there was more to come and I had no idea the next experience rock my entire world.

April 2016, I learned my son experienced something very traumatic. So many nights I cried and slept in my son's room. I had so many negative thoughts and emotions as I blamed myself, his father and paternal grandmother. I wanted to cause bodily harm to those who hurt him. I was enraged, and once again, scattered thoughts and emotions are incredibly unhealthy. I became more overprotective of him as I wanted to keep him in a bubble so that he wouldn't have to experience more pain. In all that, I realized my son has a journey of his own, and everything was right where it was supposed to be. My heart bled for my son, but I was grateful to be home and nurture him.

I discovered at that moment; quitting my job was necessary as my son needed my presence, not my presents. The Universe (God) knows what I need, and I was even more grateful for Patrick and being home.

My son's story is his story to tell, so I will not delve into his, but it is important to share how toxic my mindset and emotions were during this time as they are the beginning of any physical disease. The physical manifestation gains your attention to what is already present emotionally and spiritually. If I had known, my son would need me at home; quitting my job would have been a lot easier after learning about his experience. I'm confident I would not have been emotionally and mentally bankrupt. But, that is neither here nor there, what happened has happened as I am just delighted to share my journey to optimal health to help you heal.

Optimal health starts in your mind. According to Louis Hay (1999), we are each responsible for our experiences. Every thought we think creates our future. The point of power is always in the present moment. Everyone suffers from self-hatred and guilt. The bottom line is, I'm not good enough. It's only a thought, and thoughts can be changed. We create every so-called illness in our body. Resentment, criticism, and guilt are the most damaging patterns. Releasing resentment will dissolve even cancer. We must release the past and forgive everyone. We must be willing to begin to learn to love ourselves. Self-approval and self-acceptance in the now are the keys to positive changes. When we love ourselves, everything in our life works (Hay, 1999).

Guilt filled my mind as I blamed myself. I resented Darrell Cooper Jr as I felt betrayed by his actions. I treated him like he was my son. I hated myself for not listening to my spirit when I was guided numerous times to not allow my son back in his paternal grandmother's house. I felt ashamed, criticized myself continuously and lost all sense of being a good mom. I kept those emotions bottled up inside of me. Months passed before I released my toxic feelings and before I knew it, dis-ease and a whole lot more set up shop inside of me. My body was hijacked.

What you must understand before I move on is the body is at ease at birth; unless your mother had toxic thoughts, emotions, and behaviors or ate chemical infused food; then you will come out of the womb with a dis-eased body. However, based on our thoughts, feelings, and actions (what we ingest included), we create dis-ease in our bodies or as doctors call it, disease. I know that is hard to believe as doctors would have you think, we "catch" disease or sickness is hereditary. Well, that is all a part of the indoctrination to keep you dependent upon the healthcare and the pharmaceutical system, so the elitist maintain their lifestyles. What's more, as long as you continue to disregard your personal power, you will never know that you can heal your own body without other drugs and chemicals.

Personal power or solar plexus chakra (3rd chakra) is our willpower and governs our ability to achieve greatness and mentally understand our deepest emotions. Chakras are energetic vortexes within the human spiritual body that attracts and emits energy. We have seven within us as they as also govern the health of a specific organ. The personal power chakra controls the digestive system and its ability to digest nutrition as activated by yellow foods, clothing, etc. An inactivated or closed personal power chakra results in some of the dis-ease I experienced and discussed in this book. In order, color and location within the body are the first chakra or the root (red and tailbone). The second is the sex (pelvic area and orange). The third as discussed and the fourth is the heart (chest and green). The fifth is the third eye (between the eyes and indigo) and lastly, the crown (top of head and purple). All of the chakras represent certain emotions or energies. But for this book, I explained 3rd chakra as mine was profoundly affected. In essence, toxic emotions affect us physically. By the time the physical disease manifests, the corresponding unhealthy emotions or energy in motion has already affected the chakra.

19

Toxic emotions become embedded in our DNA. According to Dr. Stagg (2016), chronic stress and negative emotions both take their toll on the body. Relatively recent discoveries finally explain why your mind can have such broad-reaching effects on virtually every body system. We used to think this was just driven by hormones and nervous systems chemical messages. It turns out that it is much deeper than that explanation (Stagg. 2016).

Emotions of fear, frustration, and anger can result in genetic changes. Negative feelings and reactions to stress can affect your DNA through a process called epigenetic modification. Epigenetic modification means your DNA gets tagged in a way that it can completely turn on or off specific genes. For example, turning off a tumor suppressor gene could result in the proliferation of cancer cells. Your DNA contains the code for all your body proteins and enzyme systems, so no bodily function is off limits here (Stagg, 2016).

I know this to be true as after every emotionally traumatic experience in my life there was a dis-ease to follow. After sexual molestation, I criticized myself a lot with words and phrases like, *I'm worthless, I will never be good enough and I hate myself.*

According to Louis Hay, and to emphasize Dr. Stagg's scientific reasoning of negative emotions leads to disease, self-criticism leads to migraines and my goodness I had headaches that impaired my peripheral vision.

So, the information I share here is not just theory, but experience as well. I will share a few more of the mind-body disorders I experienced so that you understand that we create dis-ease in our body. About five years ago, doctors diagnosed me with Pneumonia, and during that time, I was tired and desperate to be free of old wounds; like the wound of watching my brother and his alcohol experience as he physically abused my siblings. I had a psychological fear of men that drank and never healed from the pain of watching my brother inflict so much pain on our family.

So to be married to a man who drank and became indifferent, angry and jealous reminded me of the pain that lived within.

According to Louis Hay, pneumonia stems from depression and grief and not feeling worthy of living fully. What's more, I felt stifled and desperate in my life, like I was not allowed to heal. I mean Patrick reminded me of the pain that lived deep within and being in his presence, to me, made it difficult for me to recover from that wound as he was a weekend reminder of the brother I had not forgiven. Although Patrick wasn't violent, he had no love for himself or me when he was drunk. However, the moral of this example is, I created dis-ease within my body as I harbored toxic emotions. Another example, I found myself up in the middle of the night like a zombie on a regular basis. I mean every night, I was restless, and if I did go to sleep, I would awake in the middle of the night. Doctor's diagnose habitual sleeplessness or inability to sleep as insomnia, but, according to Hay (1999), it is called fear and not trusting the process of life. Now, who would trust the process of life after knowing you have parasites and yeast eating you alive from the inside? I did not. Lastly, the hypothyroidism diagnosis three years ago was said to be hereditary and because my thyroid gland did not create enough of a thyroid hormone called thyroxine. Well, why was my magnificent body not secreting enough hormones? And what gene on my ancestor's DNA chromosome passed down to my great-grandmother, then my grandmother and then my mother or father? That doesn't make sense to me. Does that make sense to you? If dis-eases are hereditary, then every disease classified as hereditary should date all the way back to our ancestors.

According to Hay (1999) issues with the thyroid represents giving up and feeling stifled. I certainly felt smothered in the beginning years of our marriage as I was sometimes afraid to speak my mind and although Pat had his set of issues, I knew he was a good man. I just wasn't prepared for all of his toxic energy. So, I stifled myself on many occasions and more than often I gave up on our marriage.

Dr. Sarno believes that gastroesophageal reflux disease (GERD), peptic ulcers, hiatus hernia, irritable bowel syndrome (IBS), spastic colitis, esophagospasm, tension and migraine headaches, tinnitus (ringing in the ears) and most cases of prostatitis and sexual dysfunction are all mind-body disorders (2007). According to Dr. Sarno (2007), psychosomatic medicine refers explicitly to physical ailments of the mind-body; diseases that may appear to be purely physical, but which have their origin in unconscious emotions, a very different and critical medical matter. When confronting physicians with a psychosomatic disorder, they do not recognize it for what it is and almost invariably treat the symptom (Sarno, 2007). Dr. Sarno stated that the medical profession has helped to spawn epidemics of pain and other common disorders affecting the lives of Americans.

Psychosomatic disorders fall into two categories; directly induced by unconscious emotions, such as pain problems (Tension Myositis Syndrome, TMS), common gastrointestinal conditions including IBS, skin disorders, allergies and many others (Sarno, 2007). The second category is those diseases in which unconscious emotions may play a role in causation but are not the only factor. They include autoimmune disorders like rheumatoid arthritis, certain cardiovascular conditions, and cancer (Sarno, 2007).

Psychosomatic processes begin in the unconscious or subconscious, that dark unmapped, and misunderstood part of our minds first identified by Sigmund Freud. Unconscious emotions are a potent factor in virtually all physical, nontraumatic ills (Sarno, 2007). In regards to TMS, depending on the deprived tissue, the brain orders a reduction of blood flow to that specific part of the body, resulting in mild oxygen deprivation, which causes pain and other symptoms (Sarno, 2007). The purpose of psychosomatic disorders is for the unconscious mind to deliberately distract the conscious mind and divert it from what transpires in the unconscious mind. Your brain diverts you from the emotional pain by creating physical pain. The same negative emotions or pain I spoke of previously that festers and creates dis-ease before it physically manifests itself. What's more, the physical pain serves the purpose of what is called secondary gain, that is, the unconscious desire on the part of the sufferer to gain sympathy, support, and release from responsibility or arduous labor, monetary gain and so forth (Sarno, 2007).

To give you a better understanding of the mind-body disorder that falls under the category TMS let's take a look at carpal tunnel syndrome. I have experienced carpal tunnel syndrome as it was excruciating. The explanation I received from doctors was that the nerve was compressed as it passed under a ligament at the wrist and the treatment was a steroid injection or surgery. However, according to Sarno (2007), a paper published in the journal, muscle and nerve suggests that nerve function returns too rapidly after the ligament has been cut to blame compression for the disorder, and that is it more likely that local ischemia is what causes the symptoms of TMS. That finding supports the idea that carpal tunnel syndrome is a manifestation of TMS. According to Hay (1999), carpal tunnel syndrome represents anger and resentment at life's injustices. I concur as when I experienced carpal tunnel; I was pregnant and furious at being pregnant by a man that didn't want my child. Those unhealthy emotions create dis-ease as well.

Emotions are nothing but energy in motion just like serotonin, endorphins, cortisol, epinephrine and norepinephrine, lactic acid, calcium, chloride, potassium, and sodium. All of those chemicals are a source of energy. Imagine harboring negativity for years. What exactly do you think that does to the body? Serotonin is a hormone, and ninety percent is created in the gastrointestinal tract. Serotonin affects mood and social behavior, appetite and digestion, sleep, memory and sexual desire and function. Dopamine is a chemical in your brain that affects your emotions, movements and your sensations of pleasure and pain. So, if we have hormones (chemicals) that affect our mood and feelings, then how would anger, worthlessness, and sorrow affect us? If I harbor unhealthy thoughts and emotions, they will become liquefied and alter our naturally occurring hormones or chemicals in our body. So, I had to release the mental baggage as well as the emotional baggage. When we refuse to release the "stinking thinking" and unhealthy emotions, the dis-ease associated with it presents itself again. For example, twenty years ago I experienced what doctors called Psoriasis. I was twenty-five or twenty-six years young. That period was only four years after I learned I was sexually molested. I felt worthless and angry. Psoriasis presented itself on my skin. Now, metaphysically speaking, and according to Hay (1999) the skin problems represents anxiety, fear, buried guck, and feeling threatened. I obviously felt threatened as during that time I stripped for money. How can you feel safe in such a vulnerable space? What's more, I was very anxious and had a lot of buried toxic energy or guck. Psoriasis represents deadening the sense of self, fear of being hurt and refusing to accept responsibility for our feelings (Hay, 1999). I was disconnected from my soul and felt dead. I stripped, drank alcohol and smoked cigarettes. I feared pain and never allow a man to get close, so I just had sex with them. And, I refused to accept responsibility for my emotions, well, at that time, I didn't know how. Sure, I was sexually molested and blamed, but my emotions are mine. So, twenty years later, here I am. Psoriasis presented itself so that I could take a look at my emotions. If at that time, I knew the "work," I could have healed my mind, body, and soul. But I didn't, it's twenty years later, and I have released those emotional toxins that stemmed from quitting the punch clock and not having the financial means to take care of Shemar and help Patrick the way I used to.

Emotional toxins have to be released or the physical manifestation or dis-ease will re-present itself. What that also confirms is that the parasites and candida overgrowth was present then. Now that I have released the emotional and mental toxins, the physical toxins will release themselves and will not return. In essence, everything is energy, and your thoughts initiate it, your emotions intensify it, and your behaviors produce it.

I have chosen to remove all people, places, and things from my life that no longer serves me a purpose. I have learned to protect my space and energy as I make it a conscious effort to practice and maintain my new way of life. I am not a vegan as the vegan lifestyle feeds yeast and parasites. I prefer to eat some fruits, vegetables, some beans and seeds and drink high alkaline water. I may still have a piece of chicken once a week if that, but please believe, within the next 24-48 hours, I flush the leftovers out of my colon. I eat with the intent to stay healthy as I eat with the intention to maintain good energy and a positive mindset. I drink more than sixty-four ounces of water daily as I exercise regularly. I feel better than I ever have as I have no idea how forty-six is supposed to feel. I feel like a teenager some days and others like twenty-one. Life is good. I thank Mr. Parasite and Ms. Yeast for showing up when they did as my healing crisis could have very well been worse.

In essence, emotions are directly related to dis-ease or mind-body disorders. One cannot exist without the other. It's no different than disease living in an alkaline environment; it's not going to happen as they thrive in an acidic environment. Well, if your mindset and emotions are toxic or acidic, prepare for dis-ease to manifest. However, if you are present to your thoughts and feelings, you can acknowledge the negativity in the very beginning and deal with it on an emotional and mental level before it even manifests at the physical level.

We are capable of creating and manifesting whatever we focus on, negative and positive alike, and in this next chapter, you will bear witness to when your spirit speaks, the physical body speaks louder, and we need to pay attention. Most of us only pay attention to what doctors tell us as we have been brainwashed to believe they are healers, when in fact they are just as indoctrinated as everyone else. They think a pill, removing body parts and chemicals are the answers and the masses of people have fallen in the same "sucken" place. Why not explore the possibilities of healing your own body? It is habitual and conforming to say, call the doctor or go to ER. Two thousand years ago, Hippocrates, the father of medicine, stated all disease begins in the gut. If that is true, then what are doctors treating? Are they treating symptoms and if so, signs of what?

CHAPTER THREE

Burning From the Inside

Sitting at my brown kitchen table facing the balcony, I read "The Divided Mind" as my body became overwhelmed with what felt like a hot flash. Was this a symptom of menopause or was it something else? I paused and thought to myself, *was that a hot flash*? I ignored it and continued to read. I repeatedly felt that burning sensation until I was no longer able to read my book. I did some research on Google as most people would; however, my twenty-three years in health care assured me that what I felt was not a hot flash. I assessed my body looking for any other symptom that may lead me to believe I was in early menopause. From the beginning of the year, my period was on and off, but I did have one. So by this time or August 2016, I had four menstrual cycles. In order to be considered, in menopause one has to have missed their period for an entire year and that was not my case.

On and off for about fifteen minutes, the burning eventually stopped. I continued to read and went on with the rest of my day. I didn't find anything on the internet that gave me clues about what happened inside my body. A week after that appointment, I felt an itch on my tailbone. I asked my son to take a look and tell me what he saw, and then I asked him to take a picture. It appeared to be ringworm, and so I went to Walgreens and purchased some hydrocortisone. I used it for two days and by day two; there was ringworm like figure at the top of my navel area. Recall back when I previously discussed the tailbone and navel area.

Before I continue, metaphysically speaking, my spirit spoke to me at that very moment, and I did not listen. Again, recall what you read about the personal power chakra, its location, and color. Reiterating and adding more information about the personal power (solar plexus or 3rd) chakra, it is located slightly above my navel and speaks to my self-esteem, security and is the core of our personality and ego. Some people call it the solar plexus as it

27

directly relates to the Sun's energy and is our internal fireplace or our willpower. Your personal power chakra is about loving, honoring, nurturing, accepting self and understanding that inner voice that guides us. Self-acceptance and how we feel about ourselves determines what we will experience in life, relationships, business and so much more. Self-love and acceptance are the most challenging as we have all been taught to love, honor and accept external of self. Don't forget the personal power chakra also regulates metabolism and digestive processes.

A balanced personal power chakra presents itself as one who is confident, self-motivated and "on fire." When this Chakra is out of balance it presents itself in people who suffer from low self-esteem, are indecisive, and suffer from anger or control issues. Keep in mind; this chakra is our own little "fireplace" or "flame," hence the title of this chapter.

Located at the base of your spine or tailbone area, the Root (Muladhara) chakra speaks to your sense of safety. A sense of safety that includes the meeting of your emotional needs, the necessities of life or whatever you consider as your needs, as well as security as you move through life's experiences. The Root Chakra is the first Chakra and creates the foundation and opening to all other Chakras. When this Chakra is balanced, it presents itself in people who worry less and felt safe as a child. People, who didn't feel safe as a child, and without intervention, will not feel secure as adults. For instance, as a child I was sexually abused, so I didn't feel safe as a child, and after quitting my job last year, I didn't feel safe; especially without the money, I used to have. I know you might think, aren't you married? Yes, I am, however, Patrick cannot provide safety for me as that is my job and another book. The money I lacked is what I attached to my security or the five basic necessities, so in the absence of it, I felt unsafe, unstable, worthless and unsure. Can you see the connection? My Root and Personal Power Chakra were closed, and it was at the location of both of them where my first rash appeared.

After realizing those two spots were not leaving, I decided to go to the University of Chicago hospital. I made an appointment to see one of their dermatologists and upon my visit, on September 22, 2016; the doctor diagnosed the lesion on my back as Psoriasis. I was also told not to scratch, take hot baths or hot steamy showers, or the Psoriasis would spread. I was told to use the steroid ointment. The dermatologist also said the lesion in my navel area was fungal and prescribed an antifungal cream. She told me to come back in thirty days and discharged me from the doctor's office. I used the antifungal cream, and wow, the lesion atop my navel disappeared. However, the ones on my back spread in an upward position. What was weird was, each time these rashes appeared, I felt that same burning sensation hours before and suddenly had red scabs on my body. The burning came from the inside. My skin was acutely inflamed, and I knew at this time, that dermatologist misdiagnosed me. I experienced what doctors called Psoriasis when I was twenty-five years young, and that experience was nothing like this one. Over the next few weeks, my body was on fire. My torso burned like hell, and all I could do was cry.

One early afternoon in October, I sat in my black computer chair bent over in tears as I rocked back and forth. My body burned like "flame on" from Fantastic Four. Pat awoke, and the look on his face screamed pain. That moment was one of the first times he witnessed me in tears. Before this moment, I was able to bear the burning sensation. It felt like hot ants crawled all over my body. Everything hurt, underwear, washing my body, clothing, sleeping, and sex was out of the question. My body was on fire from the inside, and my skin was beet red and peeled.

"Oh my God, it burns so bad."
"What can I do? Pat asked.
"I don't know." I said as I cried, literally like a baby.
The burning at this time was unbearable, and it got worse as time passed. I had no idea what to do. The steroid ointment did absolutely nothing at all. In fact, I believed the ointment caused the explosion on my stomach, breast, back, and arms to explode.

I had no idea what happened in my body, and neither did the doctors.

"What's wrong, Ma?" Shemar asked.

I looked up at Shemar and put my head back down as I continued to cry and rock back and forth."

"Ma, it's going to be okay." Shemar kissed me on my cheek and held me as I rocked back and forth in a seated position.

"I love you Ma."

"I love you too peanut. My skin burns badly. I sobbed."

Eventually, the burning stopped, and I laid down. I lost all faith in the healthcare system; a system I spent twenty-three years serving was now just a system that practiced medicine, misdiagnosed, killed people and received compensation. During those twenty-three years, the first eight I worked as a Phlebotomist (drawing blood) and the last fifteen, I worked as a Medical Technologist. I assisted physicians in the diagnosis and treatment of diseases by performing tests on tissue, blood, and other body fluids. In fact, I helped diagnose 70% of all disease. I am also a member of the American Society of Clinical Pathologist, (ASCP). However, things became obvious to me after I left healthcare. I was determined not to go back to the doctor and take control of my health. After I walked away from healthcare, I wondered what the purpose of my education was. My Associate's in Applied Science, and my Bachelors in Health Information Management was very important to healing my body as well as understanding the system. Today, having those degrees and the amount of experience I do in healthcare was all in divine order. However, I am not sure about completing my Master's Degree as at this point in my life; traditional education interferes with my greatness. The significant part about graduate school is I can always go back.

Later that night, I attempted to sleep, but the pain and burning awoke me. I looked at the clock, and it read two-thirty in the morning. I sobered. My skin suffered, and every movement it felt like my skin peeled off. I cried like a baby. In fact, crying became an everyday thing for me. I buried my head under the cover as I didn't want Shemar to hear me. I hated for him to see me suffer. But, his senses were just as sharp as mine.

"Ma, what's wrong?"

"My skin hurts peanut. I can't sleep. It feels like my skin is peeling off. It hurts badly. I cried.

"What can I do Ma?" How can I help you? I don't like to see you cry and in pain."

Shemar eyes filled with water as he sat on my bed. He lied down and held me.

"Ma, I'm going to call Pat."

"Okay. That's fine."

"Hey, Pat."

I could hear Shemar in the living room on the phone."

"Mommy is crying. She said her skin hurts badly. She's crying like really bad Pat. Can you please come home? I don't know what to do."

"Ma, Pat wants to talks to you."

I was in so much pain that talking wasn't an option.

"Hello."

"Baby."

"I'm here."

"Oh my God, you're hurting that bad?"

"Yeah, I can't even wear my night clothes. My skin burns and hurts bad."

"Oh my, okay baby, I'm coming home. Hang in there. I love you.

Dial tone.

"Ma, is Pat coming home?"

"Yeah, he is."

"Do you want me to stay in here with you until he gets here?"

"That's fine peanut."

"Okay, I'm going to lay in the bed with you. I like being in here with you anyway."

"I know. I smiled, and so did Shemar.

Since Shemar was two years old, he always showed kindness and love to me. Whenever I was down, he was there doing whatever he could to help me feel better. And things were no different in this situation. Someday, he will make a great husband, father, and servant to the Universe.

"Hey, baby. Pat said as he leaned over and kissed my forehead."

"Hey."

"Aww, I'm so sorry. What can I do?"

"I don't know what to do." Pat immediately rubbed my body starting at my legs in an upward motion.

I cried and whimpered like a baby and for the next few months that is how life was, but the worst was yet to come.

The next afternoon I screamed, jumped up and down and ran through the house. Pat and Shemar looked at me in complete disbelief. The itch was unreachable and similar to the one you feel in the back of your throat. I cried like a baby and scratched so hard, I almost bled.

"What's wrong baby?"

"Ma, what's wrong?"

"The itch won't go away; it won't stop. I can't reach it. I screamed."

"Sh*t. What should we do?"

"I don't know." I rubbed and scratched my skin as hard as I can. It feels like something is crawling under my skin. Oh my God. What the f*ck is that? I screamed. I feel something moving!"

"Kelley, get in the shower. Let's just try some, water."

I got in the cold shower and shook my legs, arms as I cried.

"Breathe baby, just relax, and breathe."

Pat did his best to calm me down. But whatever crawled under my skin wreaked havoc on me. I was miserable, and some days I wanted to die. The burning, the pain, my skin peeling and being inflamed, not being able to wear clothing, the inability to sleep, and now this deep-rooted itch was utterly unbearable. Misery was an understatement. Day in and day out, I cried, couldn't sleep, scratched like I had fleas and burned from the inside. I continued to study and be present in my graduate classes, but it wasn't easy. I was very proud of myself for doing something I never thought I could. I maintained an 'A' average in school, coached clients, facilitated events, and was a wife and mother, through the pain, burning, itching and overall misery. I was utterly overwhelmed and wanted to give up on numerous occasions. But, being a Master Force Coach taught me better.

Being a Life Coach benefited me throughout this entire ordeal. I understood my thoughts and emotions played an essential part in my healing. So many days I had coached myself out of self-pity, the victim mindset, the why me, the anger, and overall confusion. I would've felt better if I knew what happened inside my body or if the doctors had an idea. The doctors told me not to scratch and if my skin itched to apply the prescribed cream to it.

"Patrick I have not scratched my skin, so why are these rashes spreading. They are on both sides of my stomach. Those damn doctors don't know what the hell they're talking about." I washed my skin softly in the shower.
"You're right, that doesn't make sense. Why is it spreading?"
"I don't know. Do you think it's from me using the towel to wash my body?"
"I hope not. I doubt it."
Pat stared at me with a sad and confused facial expression. He was very supportive during this entire ordeal. I love him even more today.

I was very gentle with my skin and made sure not to rub too hard or scratch. I was puzzled why if I didn't scratch how one went from the size of a nickel on my navel and the other from the size of a quarter to cover my lower back. The rash spread across my hip area, the back of my thighs, my forearms and the front of my calves. I didn't understand why the rash appeared if I wasn't scratching. I was baffled, hurt, lost, confused and angry.

Over the next ninety days or from October 1st to the end of December, I experimented with food to see if a difference would take place. For October, I removed carbohydrates, sweets, and any processed foods from my diet. I only ate meat (chicken, fish or turkey) and vegetables. Now and then I had white castles. I swear that was the worst, but my tongue certainly enjoyed it.

This change affected my son Shemar drastically as he wanted what he wanted. Patrick just went with the flow. I did all the shopping and refused to purchase anything that wasn't for my health and wellness. Shemar was highly pissed off and thought it was unfair for me to make him adjust. He missed his boxed foods like macaroni, grits, rice, Nutri-grain bars and other processed boxed foods.

Each day I avoided carbohydrates, sugar, sweets and processed foods and reflecting, I noticed how my body burned like hell in the absence. I called it "spiking." It was like my body temperature rose from 98.6 to about a one hundred and fifty. I never experienced hot flashes, but I am sure, the spiking was worse than that. It almost felt like fiery ants walked all over my body. By Thanksgiving, my entire back, stomach, the sides of my stomach, back, side and front of my legs, feet, arms, and shoulders were either covered or speckled in red and raised lesions. My body was inflamed entirely and eighty percent covered in dark rashes. I was miserable.

I was so confused about what type of clothing to wear, so I rarely went outside. If I went out, I wore tights, and that was the worst thing to wear. Polyester was the worse fabric for my skin as it felt like it ripped my skin off. Patrick decided to do some research with the information we had, and he found that cotton is the best material to wear when someone has "Psoriasis." That info was perfect.

We went to Walmart and purchased some pajamas and t-shirts so that I could at least be comfortable at home. Finally, I thought, something that doesn't hurt my skin. So many days, I wanted to stay in bed and just die. But, I pulled out every ounce of God in me and moved forward. I continued to study, visit friends and family, and maintain positivity. I was one hundred percent certain that either the doctors were just as indoctrinated as most people, or wanted to keep my insurance as a source of pay for them. Either way, I had to take control of my health. I knew everything relied on me as it was time for me to take my personal power back and heal my body. But before then, I made a few more trips to the doctor.

On November 21st I followed up with the dermatologist to examine a wart I had removed on my chest. I thought it was a mole, but it wasn't. Everything went well with the removal, and that particular area of my skin healed well. One thing about this visit that stood out was that I had a massive headache. I was in tears before the doctor came in the room.

"What's wrong dear?" The nurse's face was filled with concern as we conversed.

"My head hurts terribly."

"Do you ever have migraines?"

"Over twenty years ago and this doesn't feel anything like a migraine."

"I will be sure to mention it to your doctor before she comes in. Is everything else okay?"

"Other than dealing with this so-called Psoriasis, I'm fine."

"Okay, your doctor will be in momentarily. I hope you feel better."

"Okay, thank you."

I held my head as tears flowed down my face. This headache was worse than a migraine. What the hell is going on? Why does my head hurt so badly? Maybe it is just stress from dealing with this skin issue. I thought. Patrick was always there. Right beside me holding my hand and comforting me.

"Hi Kelley, how are you feeling? My nurse told me you have a terrible headache."

"Yes, I do. I cried."

"Well, let me examine the surgical area, and we can send you over to ER.

"Okay."

"Everything looks fine. Have you had any issues with this area since the removal of the wart?"

"No, I have not."

"Okay, well it looks good. I'm going to call over to the ER department and let them know you're coming. Do you want me to get you a wheelchair?"

"No, I can walk."

"Baby, just let them get you a wheelchair." Pat intervened.

"I can walk Pat."

"Okay then, take care, Kelley."

"Thanks, doctor."

Pat and I walked over to triage, and everything in me told me just go home as I knew all they would do is offer me a pill. And I was right. After talking with the ER doctors, their solution was to take a pill. They gave me a prescription, and I tossed it in the garbage. Before Pat and I could make it to the car, my headache miraculously disappeared.

"It's gone, Pat."

"Your headache is gone?."

"Yeah, it's gone."

"Wow, what was that about?

"I don't know, but I'm glad it's gone. Thank God or the Universe."

"I'm glad you feel better baby. "

"Me too.

"Well, when we get home, you lie down and get some rest."

I spent twenty-three years in an industry that practiced medicine, treated symptoms, removed body parts and pushed chemicals and toxins into the human body and somehow got it confused with healing. Pharmaceutical drugs kill more people than street drugs. A recent analysis published in the Journal of the American Medical Association stated that 128,000 Americans die each year as a result of taking prescribed medications – or nearly five times the number of people killed by overdosing on prescription painkillers and heroin. According to the National Institute, the U.S. government does not track death rates for every drug. However, the National Center for Health Statistics at the

Centers for Disease Control and Prevention does collect information on many of the more commonly used drugs. In 2015, the number of deaths from all drugs was less than half of the deaths by prescribed medications. How astonishing is that? Healthcare drugs kill more people than street drugs, and now is the time for us to take control of our health and heal our bodies.

We were born into a world that taught us to relinquish our power or our ability to heal ourselves. Education, religion, the food and drug administration (FDA) and the healthcare systems are the main culprits that we relinquish our personal power. The educational system taught us to rely on their educational programs to obtain a job and produce income. While we punch the clock and work a job (Just over broke) we move further and further away from our divine purpose or the reason we were born. What's more, we lose a sense of belief in self, and I don't mean our ability to find a job; I mean our divine right to create what we desire and live in and on purpose. We become extremely reliant upon the job market to assist us in living just as we did during slavery. Many of us live paycheck to paycheck and have only enough money to make sure bills are paid, food is in the refrigerator, gas is in our cars and can take the occasional vacation, and the "system" would have it no other way. The same programs you studied to acquire your job and make money, was created by the same system that created the medical doctor program. What makes you think, their program is any different as the bottom line is making money? Traditional healthcare has never been about healing, and it never will be.

The religious system taught us to rely on an external God or believe in a white Jesus that apparently does not exist. Accepting or depending on this white Jesus to save us, is the death of us. God, the divine, the infinite or whatever you choose to call the source is within all life, and that includes animals and insects. Somehow we were brainwashed into believing dead energy (animal products) is acceptable for a live body to ingest. You're probably wondering what the system has to so with our health? Everything, however, I will share that later, so just keep reading.

The more we believe what the Bible tells us about meat, the more we indoctrinate our health and wellness. There was no such thing as humans eating animals until the European man lived in caves. Once the Europeans were released from caves and gained control over the world, meat and animal organs, processed foods, chemicals, artificial colors (food coloring) and flavor, and smoked foods became popular. Food became a science as the rest is history and now we live to eat instead of eating to live. Anything produced and approved by the FDA creates a profit for them and dis-ease and a slow death for us. However by popular demand, blood and starch are not even close to what's killing us.

The healthcare system taught us that disease is hereditary; we 'catch' disease, we need a pill to 'fix' us, we need to remove body parts to heal and so many more lies that encourage a slow death. Relying on practicing doctors to heal us is like relying on a rattlesnake to ignore your presence. The father of medicine said two thousand years ago; all disease begins in the gut. So, why are doctors treating symptoms? Why do we have a hospital department for every organ or system in the body? Why are doctors giving us pills for diabetes, high cholesterol, heart disease, cancer, lupus and so many other dis-eases? Why? Because they get paid to prescribe medicine or shall I say "kickbacks." Doctors also bill your insurance for all dis-ease they diagnose.   For each disease diagnosed there is specific information that determines the reimbursement. For instance, diabetes may require a certain length of stay if the patient becomes ill, routine blood draws, use of band-aids, sheets, gauze, food and any other service needed during the hospital stay or visit. With that, the system decides how much to bill the patient. Now, if all dis-ease starts in the gut, why are we not healing the gut with hydrotherapy or colon cleanse, probiotics, essential oils, detoxing elimination channels, plant-based diets, exercise, and rest? Why are doctors not focusing on the gut?

Have you ever wondered why insurance doesn't cover holistic healers like health and wellness coaches, functional and integrative doctors and alternative medical doctors? Health and wellness coaches and the other homeopathic healers treat the whole body and not just symptoms. When you treat the entire body, it results in a healthy body. Can you imagine where healthcare would be if we focused on healing the whole body or the source of dis-ease or the gut? Bankrupt.

Eighty percent of the immune system is in your gut and protected by a lining that acts as a barrier to your gut's toxic environment. If that fence is damaged, (leaky gut) like mine was, the toxins compromise your immune system, and that is when the inflammation or autoimmune response begins. What's more, the body is no longer capable of absorbing the nutrients it needs to maintain health or protect it from harmful chemicals or products. How do I know? That is what I experienced after my immune system became compromised as my gut filled with every toxic product and chemical you can imagine and forty-five years of it. It took me forty-five, well, now, forty-six years to realize that the FDA lied about what is good for the human body to ingest.

According to the FDA and the food pyramid we are supposed to have two-three servings of meat, poultry, and fish, six to eleven servings of bread, cereal, rice and pasta, and two to three servings of milk, yogurt, and cheese. What's more, the fruit and vegetable servings are one three to five servings of vegetable and two to four servings of fruit. Why do the animal products and processed foods outweigh the fruits and vegetables? Because the more meat and processed foods you eat, the sicker you become, thereby sending you straight to the hospital, receiving a pill and praying to your external God and relinquishing your personal power.

What do the FDA, religion, healthcare and the education system have to do with my health and wellness or yours? They are constituents of the "system." The same system that makes billions and trillions of dollars telling us to tithe, and pay the building fund is the same system that programmed us to celebrate with a thirty dollar steak fused together with blood platelets and drink alcohol. As we eat chemically (artificial or natural flavors) infused boxed foods, we sit in a classroom that forces us to behave like robots and only repeat what we have learned and without any creativity. Where are our independent thoughts and personal power? I will tell you.

The creative human has been indoctrinated to believe everything mainstream throws our way, and we are now robotic and programmed never to ask questions.

So again, you ask what the "system" has to do with taking my power back and healing myself. We have been taught to relinquish our power to those external forces and never honestly see the infinite possibilities that are within us. Your personal power is the center of your abilities to do anything you choose and create whatever you desire, and that includes heal your body if you have the proper information and beliefs.

In fact, part of me wanted the doctors to be correct about the diagnosis of Psoriasis as that was an easy fix, from what I remember. I remember being diagnosed with Psoriasis when I was twenty-five years old, but I don't remember burning the way that I did. I used hydrocortisone cream, and it went away in about three weeks. I had many questions as I compared twenty years ago.

What is the difference?
Why does it burn?
Why are the rashes larger than before?
Why did the steroid cream not work?
Why is my skin pealing?
Why does my skin hurt?
Why is the itch so deep?
Why can't I reach the itch?

I was not convinced that Psoriasis was the proper diagnosis. Everything I experienced was far more detrimental than my previous experience with Psoriasis. However, I did a lot of research on skin disorders and learned there was a deeper problem. I even I wrote a blog on Psoriasis and shared it with the public. I have removed it since that time. The information I found was more profound than the skin, literally, and would take longer than three weeks to heal. I decided to revisit the doctors as this "rash" spread and got worse. I wanted the doctors to confirm what I found as they only made another diagnosis.

Self-Diagnosis

Thanksgiving arrived, and I cooked dinner for Patrick and Shemar, but I visited my sister's house for dinner. My sisters were very kind as they rubbed shea butter or lotion on my back when needed. My spirit told me not to eat anything served at my sister's house. But, of course, I was hardheaded. I had some greens, a spoonful of macaroni, some salad, and turkey. The day after Thanksgiving my body was worse. I was in tears and running through the house like a madman. I knew something was making its way into my bloodstream, but I wasn't sure what it was. I was miserable. I blamed the GMO food as I regretted eating the foods my sister cooked. However, blame was of no importance as I am aware of my creative abilities. My focus was to find a solution and that I did. So many days, I wanted to stay in bed and just die. But, I pulled out every ounce of God in me and kept moving forward. I continued to study, visit friends and family, and maintain positivity. I was one hundred percent certain that either the doctors were just as indoctrinated as most people or wanted to keep my insurance as a source of pay for them. Either way, I had to take control of my health. I knew everything relied on me as it was time for me to take my personal power back and heal my body.

Right before Christmas, I decided to see an acupuncture doctor. My entire body was inflamed, red, burning and I was miserable. I drove to Naperville, Illinois and received the acupuncture treatment.

"Open your mouth and stick out your tongue."

Dr. Lee was a kind lady.

"You have a lot of heat in your body. Your tongue is like fire, fire."

I wasn't exactly sure what she meant, but I certainly made the connection of something caused my body to produce so much heat and inflammation. I never had acupuncture before, but Dr. Lee did a good job explaining the process with her limited English.

"Your skin has four layers of energy, and there is a distraction within all layers. The acupuncture will restore your energy, but you will have to come back and take tea."

"Okay. What tea?

"Herbs, to help clean out your blood. You should have come sooner."

What's in my blood?"

"I'm not sure, but it's causing a lot of heat. Your tongue is like red, that means fire, heat, hot. Go ahead and undress from the waist down and pull your shirt up. You can keep your panties on."

I undressed, and Dr. Lee looked at my body.

"You should have come sooner."

My eyes filled with water as I was very emotional and sad at this time. I wanted to heal. I wanted answers as I was tired of suffering. Dr. Lee placed needles in my stomach (near my navel) my calves, forehead, arms, and legs. She turned on some soft music.

"Please close your eyes and relax."

She also had some gadget that produced more heat placed over the needles. I didn't understand that, but I trusted she knew what she was doing. Pat sat in a chair near the window. He was always right there, supporting and comforting me. Tears flowed down the side of my face as I laid on the bed on top of a white sheet. I was cold, but eventually, felt relaxed.

"Relax baby. You're going to be okay."

Pat came over and wiped my tears.

"Just relax."

It didn't matter what I needed. If Pat had to take off work, he did. During my research and minutes before my acupuncture appointment, I stumbled across a website that discussed acupuncture and Psoriasis. I read about how much heat is produced within the body as I read the toxicity levels that created the heat. But, there was no mention of what caused the heat or toxicity. I was happy with the information I read but somewhat sad as I still had no answer to what caused the heat, inflammation, damage to my skin, and the pain. I decided to give acupuncture a try as nothing else worked.

The treatment lasted about forty-five minutes and cost seventy-five dollars. I felt some relief, but not enough to heal my body. I didn't expect one treatment to cure me, but I sought something to provide the comfort. I also purchased some blood cleansers. The pills were small, circular and black. I had to take six pills a day for eleven days, and after about a week of using them, I didn't feel the burning. I was happy. I felt relief and was excited to go back and purchase the herbal teas. The teas were blood cleansing teas. At that moment, I realized something caused my body to "flame on" from the inside. I realized there was something in me, but what?

"You come back in one week to get your herbs."

"Okay. Thank you, Dr. Lee."

I never went back to get the tea, but I did purchase some nicotine patches. I used the patches for four days, and on December twenty-fourth, 2016, Pat and I sat on the floor on a pile of blankets and sheets and watched movies. Sitting on the couch wasn't an option. I removed the patch as I didn't want anything else going in my blood.

"Pat, if there is something in my blood causing all this inflammation, what is the difference in the nicotine delivered to my bloodstream from this patch. I don't want anything else going in blood."

I smoked a cigarette after I removed the patch. I knew I would, but I had more than enough reason to quit. In fact, I had a cigarette with an X through it on my vision board. I desired to release the addiction to smoking. I smoked my last salem light one hundred on December 24, 2016, and haven't looked back. I never thought after thirty years of smoking cigarettes; I would finally quit. I had no desire to smoke another cigarette. Instantaneously, I became grateful for this experience. I was no longer sad, angry or confused. I realized this was all for my highest good and not my demise. I realized something more significant was to come as this experience like all of mine, were higher than me and not really about me. Immediately, I thanked the Universe and shifted my paradigm. I went from unhappy, sad and miserable, to joyful, positive and hopeful. December 24 changed my life immediately, physically, emotionally and mentally. However, some days were still a struggle.

While researching skin disorders, I stumbled across Dr. Axe's website and discovered that Leaky Gut causes skin disorders. According to Dr. Axe, Leaky Gut is Intestinal Permeability. A possible cause of leaky gut is increased intestinal permeability or intestinal hyperpermeability. That happens when tight junctions in the gut, which control what passes through the lining of the small intestine, don't work correctly. That could let substances leak into the bloodstream (Dr. Axe). In lay terms, tears or holes in your gut or small intestine. The small intestine is the part of the intestines where ninety percent of digestion and absorption of nutrients and minerals from food occurs.

After reading the information found on Dr. Axe's website, I made a self-diagnosis of Leaky Gut as some of the symptoms listed were bloating, fatigue, joint pain, headaches, weight gain, syndrome X digestive problems, food sensitivities, thyroid conditions, skin issues like rosacea and acne. Every website I researched said the same thing. There was a correlation between leaky gut and skin disorders. But, there was a lot more than even these holistic doctors weren't discussing.

If leaky gut was my diagnosis and considered to be tears or hole in the small intestine, then the two thousand four hundred milligrams of Motrin doctors prescribed me for migraines when I was seventeen caused them. What I do know after spending twenty-three years in healthcare is that Motrin or non-steroidal anti-inflammatory drugs (NSAID's) causes ulcers. Doctor's at Jackson Park hospital diagnosed me with a peptic ulcer in my junior year of high school. The interesting part is that I experienced all of the symptoms of leaky gut except syndrome X. As far as the digestive problems are concerned, I have experienced irritable bowel syndrome, gastroesophageal reflux disease, inflammatory bowel disease, diarrhea, and constipation. I was diagnosed with hypothyroidism four years ago, and prior to that diagnosis, I gained twenty-five pounds. I was diagnosed with having at least twenty five food sensitivities after having my blood tested. My knee joints hurt continuously and I was always tired and fatigue. Lastly, the reason this book exists, the doctors at the University of Chicago hospital diagnosed me with Psoriasis, Pityriasis Rosacea, and Lichen Planus.

I was somewhat relieved to have an idea of what destroyed my skin and made me feel so sick. I reflected back on how many of these symptoms I experienced and realized I must have had Leaky Gut since I was at least seventeen years old. That is a long time, I thought to myself, so it is no wonder my body fell apart. I followed all of the instructions Dr. Axe shared on his website as I purchased all of the supplements. My Uncle Jimmy was very instrumental and supportive during this time. If Pat or I didn't have the money to buy my supplements, Uncle Jimmy came to the rescue.

He was more than willing to loan me the money as I was and am very grateful for my mother's brother. I made monthly trips to the Whole Foods store in Orland and became a regular where many of the cashiers and floor employees knew who I was.

There was one gentleman in particular, and his name was Bill. He was very kind and even when my skin looked horrible; Bill found it in his heart to listen and help me find my supplements. I shared a few words with him two weeks before he resigned from the Whole Foods Store.

Some of the supplements I took were L-Glutamine, Licorice, Milk Thistle, 5000 IU of vitamin D, collagen, and HCL. However, none of those products worked with a toxic colon. How would they be digested and absorbed? I used psyllium husk to clean my colon and did that for about two weeks before using the supplements. I didn't realize I had so much stool in me as the turds were nearly nine inches long and pretty think. They reminded me of when I was a child as I was amazed at how something so long could exit a small person. But understanding the size of the colon, it wasn't abnormal. After the two weeks expired, I released about ten pounds of waste from my body.

During the supplements, I decided to avoid meat and any starchy food as I watched some of my skin go from beet red and purple raised rashes and scaly to covered in dark brown and black raised patches. I was happy. I knew the hyperpigmentation would clear as long as I did what I was supposed to do. In fact, since October, my body has been on the road to recovery. I included green juices to my diet and at least two a day. I continued to exercise to assist in the peristalsis (intestinal muscle movement). I drank more water than I ever drank or so I thought and was determined to heal my body without any traditional doctors. However, I went back to the University of Chicago Hospital on December 19th.

I saw the dermatologist and received another misdiagnosis. I was so hurt and upset. Dark, raised spots covered my body and were apparent to the naked eye.

"The new rashes are Pityriasis. What have you been using on your skin?"

The doctor scanned my entire body as I stood naked.

"I use shea butter with essential oils like tea tree and lavender."

"Don't use that on your skin. It can cause a flare up or damage your skin. Use the steroid we gave you."

"It doesn't work and is it a possibility that I have leaky gut?"

"No, but you have to stop drinking alcohol."

"I haven't been drinking." I frowned at the doctor.

She stood there next to the sink with this dumb look on her face.

"Well, something is causing you to break out."

"You're the doctor, you should know."

"I've researched leaky gut and Psoriasis, and there is a correlation."

"Leaky gut has nothing to do with skin disorders. However, it can be autoimmune. I'm going to schedule you for some blood test."

47

"Are you sure? How do you know for certain that it's not leaky gut, food particles or something else leaking into my bloodstream?"

That doctor blew off my question as she never answered it with other than, let's draw some blood. That blood test didn't take place until February 8, 2017. I refused to go back to that hospital anytime soon. University of Chicago hospital is the same hospital I sued for medical malpractice and won as they killed my mother in surgery. I was discharged and received a list of chemicals to put on my skin, but was told not to use natural essential oils and shea butter. The dermatologist recommended Vaseline petroleum jelly, Aquaphor ointment, Cetaphil moisturizing cream, Cerave cream and Eucerin cream. Along with that, the doctors prescribed Vanicream cream and Amlactin cream. She also recommended Neutrogena oil-free facial moisturizer with SPF, Cetaphil facial moisturizer, Cerave facial cream AM (with SPF) or PM (no sun protection) and Eucerin sensitive skin facial lotion.

There weren't any rashes on my face, and I certainly wasn't going to prepare for any. I was so happy my face was clear. I left the doctor's office once again feeling disappointed and angry. However, I went to Walgreen to purchase some cream. I was so desperate to heal my skin. I still had no idea of what happened on the inside, so I focused on the outside or, my skin and what was visible. I purchased the Cerave, and it burned, so I took it back to Walgreens. I went to Mariano's and bought some Aquaphor. Although the Aquaphor didn't heal my skin, it did provide some relief and extra moisture. I was able to sit down and not hurt the back of my legs. I even used Vaseline for a few weeks, but nothing seemed to help the itch or pain. The burning resolved, or at this time, I had no more "flare-ups." I was indeed happy to get the burning sensation resolved. I noticed when I experienced the "flare ups," the next day, I had new rashes.

I also noticed since I changed my diet to a plant-based diet, I felt a lot better than before. But again, the itching was never ending and a complete pain in my ass. In the wee hours of

December 26th, I cried and scratched persistently. My skin itched severely. I did not know what to do. I thought about going to Walgreens to purchase Benadryl, but I knew it would mask the real issue or whatever that was.

"Pat, I can't stop itching." I cried

"Do you want to go to ER?"

"Yes, I do."

I needed something. I wanted answers and the itch to stop. Pat drove to the University of Chicago hospital, and two ER doctors examined me.

"Kelley Porter Turner." A male nurse called my name.

Pat and I got up and walked to triage nursing station where I explained the diagnosis of Psoriasis and Pityriasis Rosacea. The triage nurse took my vitals and sent me back to the waiting room. I itched like hell, and wanted to peel my skin off my body. My skin was reddish-purple, scaly, grey, black, and itchy, and in so much pain. I sat in the waiting room rocking back and forth as Pat rubbed my back. I cried, and the few people who were there stared at me.

"Kelley Porter Turner."

"I'm right here."

I got up, and two doctors told me to follow them to a room not located in the ER patient room. I pulled my pants down and my shirt up. Both of their eyebrows rose with their eye wide open.

"I was told I have Psoriasis and Pityriasis Rosacea by the doctors here. I don't know what to do. The itch is driving me crazy."

"Your skin is extremely damaged especially around your hip areas."

I turned around so they could see my back and they were just as shocked. I cried

"What can you all do to help me?"

"I'm sorry, but if the dermatologist couldn't do anything, I'm not sure what we can. We're only emergency room doctors."

"Okay, well is there anything you can give me for the itch? I can't sleep, and I just want to go to sleep. I cried."

"Sure. We can prescribe something that will stop the itch."

"Thank you."

"Go ahead and get dressed and we will see you back in the waiting room."

Pat and I went back to the waiting room and sat for about fifteen minutes.

"Mrs. Turner."

"Yes." I stood up and walked towards the doctors.

They handed me a prescription written out for Benadryl.

"Thank you."

"You're welcome, and I hope you feel better."

That was it. A pill used to suppress the release of histamines in my body. But why was my body releasing so many histamines?

As a medical technologist, and understanding hematology (the study of blood) a part of my education was to understand the function of white blood cells, (WBC's). Basophils release histamines during allergic or inflammatory responses. A high basophil count can also assist in diagnosing infection, inflammation, leukemia, or an immune system disorder.

The release of basophils helps to control inflammation, and the count is unusually high during parasite infections as they also help stop substances or other foreign materials from harming the body.

Increased eosinophils represent parasitic infections and other conditions. My question is when I first went to the doctor with Psoriasis symptoms, why did the doctors request an cbc (complete Blood Count) that which includes an eosinophil and basophil count. Doctor's describe Psoriasis as a skin disease marked by red, itchy, scaly patches. The red represented inflammation (swelling, tenderness, and infection); the itch represents healing, allergies, creepy crawly, and the flaky patches was just damaged skin. So, why treat a skin disorder when the answer is in the blood? Doctors are trained to handle symptoms and not the whole body.

From this point, I focused on healing the Leaky Gut, but my spirit led me to continue with my research. I researched Leaky

Gut and foods to eat and stumbled across another holistic doctor that focused on recipes to heal your gut. Dr. Amy Meyers offered a free recipe book on four things. Her book also mentioned the same supplements that Dr. Axe spoke about on his website. I was excited. I knew I was on the right path and healing was within my reach. According to Dr. Meyers (2015), nine signs indicate Leaky Gut. Dr. Meyers believe that as your immune system becomes more stressed or compromised, it is less able to attack pathogens and invaders with accuracy. Instead, the immune system eventually attacks your bodies owns tissue. I disagree. How can the human body become so stupid, angry and confused that it attacks itself? That doesn't make sense to me as the body only strikes foreign objects that present themselves in the bloodstream, unless, those foreign objects mimic our protein molecules.

The information I have as well as the proof will prove to you and the world that even autoimmune disorder really doesn't exist.

Dr. Meyer's nine signs that indicate leaky gut surround your organs systems. In regards to your skeletal system, if you have osteopenia or osteoporosis there's a chance you have Leaky Gut. The last time I checked, doctors said bone issues were due to lack of cow milk or vitamin D deficiency. In fact, cow milk causes the body and bones to break down. The FDA approved thousands or maybe millions of somatic cells to be in milk and marketed as safe. According to Chemometec (2017), the somatic cell count (SCC) is used as an indicator of the quality of milk. If the number of somatic cells in the milk exceeds certain limits, the milk cannot be sold for human consumption. The accurate measurement of the concentration of somatic cells in milk is critical. Also, milk yields tend to decline when somatic cell counts increases, increasing the need for precise monitoring of the concentration of somatic cells in the milk (Chemometec, 2017).

What are somatic Cells? Somatic Cells are cells of the body that is composed of tissue, organs, and parts of that individual other than a germ cell. What does that mean? According to my

American Society of Clinical Pathologist (ASCP) certificate, somatic cells include leukocytes or white blood cells (WBC); therefore cow WBC's are present in cow milk. That means you are drinking cow's blood when you drink cow's milk. Chemometec (2017) stated most of the somatic cells in milk are leukocytes. Leukocytes are white blood cells and responsible for protecting us from pathogens or other disease producing bacteria or viruses. When white blood cells are activated, they create a pus or mucus-like substance. How does this affect the human body? According to my twenty-three years in healthcare, my degree in Medical Laboratory Science and Health Information Management, excess mucus in the body produces dis-ease. In fact, every specimen I analyzed as a Medical Laboratory Technician (MLT), I witnessed large amounts of mucus. Those samples included pleural (chest) fluid, synovial (knee) fluid, cerebral spinal fluid (CSF), vaginal, throat, feces, and other body fluids. So, if cow milk contains white blood cells, how do you think their mucus is affecting us?

Cow milk has been said to drain calcium from your bones to neutralize the acidity. What's more cow milk is made to turn a 63 pound baby calf into a 600 pound cow in eight months. There are 35 hormones and 11 growth factors in cow's milk and one of them has been linked to breast and prostate cancer. Cow milk is also high in saturated fat and cholesterol. So why are you drinking it? You are still drinking cow milk because the FDA said it was good for you; *Got Milk, Got Disease*. Drink coconut or almond milk. Does a calf drink human milk? No. I wonder why. Have you ever wondered why melted cheese is like slime? Well, take a look at mucus.

Dr. Meyers stated that when dealing with the brain if people suffer from anxiety, depression or brain fog, they have leaky gut. To a certain degree, I agree, however, in my current experience, not theory, brain fog, anxiety, and depression is a lot deeper than leaky gut. What exactly is in the colon that makes its way to our brain? What chemicals does the colon send to our brain?

When suffering from digestive dis-ease like bloating, constipation, diarrhea, weight loss, and fat malabsorption, you are suffering from leaky gut (Dr. Meyers, 2015). With that, I can hypothetically assume that everyone has or at one point suffered from leaky gut. When it comes to hormones, Dr. Meyers stated that if you suffer from irregular periods, premenstrual syndrome (PMS), perimenopause or menopausal systems you have leaky gut. Other doctors will tell you that some of those conditions are age-related. If you have frequent colds, the flu, infections, joint or muscle pain, or autoimmune disorders, Dr. Meyers believes you have leaky gut. I have experienced all of them and told it was the weather, another person, old age-related, or unknown etiology.

Metabolism, excess weight, obesity and diabetes indicate leaky gut. Why are doctors telling us that Diabetes is hereditary? Both my parents had diabetes, and I do not. Only two of my siblings experienced diabetes, and that was because of their diet and obesity. No disease is hereditary. That has to be the stupidest suggestion I have ever heard. Have you ever wondered why you cannot lose weight after exercise and diet? Well, if you are robbed of your nutrition, whether it is Parasites or Leaky Gut, cells and organs will not function correctly resulting in the inability to metabolize foods leading to weight gain, or the failure to release weight.

Of the nine signs that indicate leaky gut, the one thing that stood out to me was the dis-ease listed under the "gut." Under the gut section, Dr. Meyers lists parasites, small intestinal bacterial overgrowth (SIBO) and yeast overgrowth (candida). Is it a possibility that the parasites and yeast are responsible for all dis-ease in the human body and everything else is an addition to or accelerator of the dis-ease? It indeed is a possibility and based on the worms and yeast I released from my body; I am 100% sure parasites and yeast overgrowth is the cause for all dis-ease.

You might wonder why I hyphenate the word "disease." The body is at "ease" when we are born. However, similac from the so-called Women's, Infant and Children program (WIC) was nothing but a set up to make us sick. Imagine a newborn drinking a can of sugar as that all similac is. Sugar feeds yeast, so if mom doesn't breastfeed, her baby will not receive passive immunity or antibodies from her breast. Colostrum is loaded with antibodies and when a baby lack antibodies, imagine what that yeast will do to the body. Imagine a baby drinking similac (a can of sugar) for nine months, while feeding the yeast. By the time that baby is nine months; the yeast has already taken over. And do not think for one minute the government or the system did not plan this. If you are a parent, reflect on how sick your child was. Did he or she suffer from skin issues, diarrhea, constipation, fever, pain, crying and sick for unknown reasons? Think about how often your toddler was sick with stomach pain, itchy rashes, white tongue or oral thrush. Oral thrush is a fungal infection. How and why? We have been ill from day one, and all we have done is get older and sicker. Why does a baby have a fungal infection in her mouth? Yeast is in our mouths for protective reasons. So how does it overgrow? It needs food. What does a baby drink? Babies in America drink similac. Don't think for one minute, the elitist like Rockefeller and his friends from the AMA and other corporations hasn't studied candida albicans and intestinal worms. How do you think the "Quacks" knew how to kill parasites? They tested on humans just as we are guinea pigs today. Have you heard of the Tuskegee study of untreated syphilis? Now, I want you to think about the disease you suffer from today. Does your dis-ease(s) sound anything like what your child experienced? Mine does. Lastly, what is similac?

What's in that can that's free to moms and especially in the black communities? Think about that. Why do we need to feed a baby some garbage from a can when we have breast that feeds our babies precisely what they need. Have you ever wondered why we breastfed our slave masters, white babies? Think about that. They knew the importance of breastfeeding. And the moment the European put a can in our face with some cheese, cereal, and eggs and said it's free, we neglected our babies and fed them a can of sugar, some pus, starch and more sugar. Now here we are today, sick and slowly dying, and from birth while making the elite richer. Have you ever thought about why everybody has the same dis-ease?

My son's body broke out when he was nine years old. The rash covered forty percent of his body. He scratched until he bled and doctors had no idea what it was. His pediatrician blamed the new suit I bought him and then said it was Pityriasis Rosea. To this day, my son's skin has not completely healed, and he is 16. There are still a few marks left on his back. In essence, doctors can blame leaky gut, but your gut didn't just decide to leak one day. Something had to penetrate the barrier. Something had to make the walls of your intestines weak. I can guarantee yeast is culprit along with other toxins, such as ingesting blood (animal products) and starch (rice, pasta, bread, boxed foods), and let's not forget emotions toxins and "stinkin thinkin."

Candida albicans start out as small buds, circular like structures, however, after yeast is fed sugar, and starchy foods over a period of time, yeast become hyphae. Hyphae look like a tree with branches under the microscope. At that point, the yeast is strong and pathogenic. I can guarantee it is the overgrowth of yeast that penetrates the lining of the small intestines causing permeability and toxic waste products and bacteria to "leak" through the intestines and surge the bloodstream. Once the parasite and yeast are free from the gut, guess where they can run, hangout and hide; your skin, lungs and even your brain. Believe it or not, I have felt them in my skin, head and attempt to run up my lungs as I gagged.

Dr. Amy Meyers and Dr. Axe both agree as it relates to the 4R approach. Remove, Replace, Reinoculate and Repair. What are we removing? Removing inflammatory foods and allergens is essential. What foods replaced the inflammatory foods? You replace the inflammatory or allergen foods with foods from the earth and not laboratory foods. What are we reinoculating? You reinoculate the body with probiotics. Probiotics are "good" bacteria that help maintain the 80/20 rule. The 80/20 rule states that as long as we maintain 80% good bacteria in the gut and

20% bad bacteria, our bodies will maintain optimal health. Lastly, when are we repairing? We repair the tears in our gut that allows toxins, undigested foods, and other particles to cross over into the immune section of our gut.

How does leaky gut cause so many dis-eases in the body? What exactly is in the gut that makes us sick? As mentioned earlier, eighty percent of the immune system is in your gut and protected by a lining that acts as a barrier to your gut's toxic environment. If that barrier is damaged, your immune system is compromised, and that is when the inflammation, autoimmune response or creation of dis-ease begins. What this means is humans do not "catch" dis-ease, we create them. We have been taught and programmed to believe that we "catch" disease. What if you were responsible for all the dis-ease you have ever experienced? What if you created the dis-ease in your body? Doesn't that mean you can un-create it and not have to rely on doctors to prescribe you a pill? What does that say about your personal power? You can heal your own body if you accept the fact that you are responsible for what goes in your mouth. In essence, leaky gut is a huge part of healing the body, and in my case, Psoriasis, Pityriasis Rosacea, and Lichen Planus are all symptoms of something bigger and broader than leaky gut. My skin; that is an organ, suffered more than any other organ in my body.

The hyperpigmentation and fears of what people would think of me almost led me to depression. Many days I didn't want to be seen, and wanted to die.

But, today, I rise and stand firm as the hyperpigmentation has empowered and elevated my life in so many ways. I am beyond grateful. This experience has transformed my entire being. Things I thought I could not do, I can do today. I am one hundred percent certain that all things that occur in our daily life are for our highest good. I am free from the bondage of looks, vanity, perfection, societal acceptance, and ideal beauty. I am beauty and so are you.

CHAPTER FIVE

Lichen Planus Diagnosis

I decided to visit the Gynecologist, and my thoughts were right. I was not in early menopause as I would have had to miss a period for twelve months consecutively. That confirmed what I learned from reading Dr. Meyers information on her website. I blamed everything on Leaky Gut. But, what happened inside my body? How was my gut connected to missed periods, hypothyroidism and all other dis-ease? What was the connection? I refused to give up as I asked the angels to guide me to the information I needed to heal my body.

By the beginning of February, I was back to square one; burning, itching, blistering, lack of sleep and complete misery. I cried more, prayed, meditated, and never stopped exercising and studying for my Master's Degree. I suffered drastically and worse than the first time around. I wasn't sure what I did or what I was supposed to do. More than half of my body was inflamed. My entire back, thighs, the back of my legs, the back of my arms, elbows, feet, and the back of my calves were inflamed. The rashes were raised, red and very tender. What's more, I noticed a bald spot in the back of my head and that broke my heart. It took me two years to grow my hair from a very short fade to having two long french braids. When I was seven years old, my sister permed my hair, and after that day, the only way I knew to comb my hair was with two french braids. I never learned how to take care of my hair without a perm. I was in a space where I wanted to experiment with my natural hair, and for two years, I combed it, twisted, braided it, and wore ponytails, double strand twist, and so much more. I was thrilled to embrace my kinky, thick hair as I was excited to comb it daily. It was not a chore to me, but an opportunity to embrace my full blackness. Day after day, my hair fell out. I stood in the mirror with a handheld mirror and looked at the back of my head. That one bald spot had spread. *Well, I refuse to suffer and watch my hair fall out, so I'm cutting it off.* I thought.

"Bae, some more of my hair has fallen out. Come and look."

"Awww man. It sure did."

"I'm not even going to bother with the doctors as all they're going to say is that its alopecia."

"So, what are you going to do?"

"I'm going to cut it."

"Wow. It took you two years to grow your hair, and now you have to cut it off."

I wanted to cry, but I was happy that I had the opportunity to care for my natural hair and watch it grow. I even had two ponytails. I shaved my hair back down to the low fade, and not less than a week later the entire back of my head was hairless. I was forced to go bald. And again, that didn't affect me as I wore a low fade for over ten years before allowing my hair to grow. Shemar walked in the bathroom.

"Ma, I love your hair, it's so beautiful. I think I'm going to let my hair grow."

"Really peanut. I smiled from ear to ear. I am so happy to hear you say that. (My eyes filled with tears.) It is an honor to hear you embrace the natural black woman. Embracing my hair means you not only embrace yours, but you embrace being black, and that brings me joy."

"Yeah momma, I'm sorry you have to cut it. But you will be okay. You're used to having a low cut."

"You're right."

Hearing my son embrace my kinky, thick hair and what white America deemed as nasty or ugly, was the best compliment. I never imagined that coming from a fifteen-year-old. My son attends school with predominately White or Hispanic kids, so there's not a lot of natural hair exposed to him as most of the melanated girls have perms. Furthermore, TV rarely portrays a black woman with natural hair as it is usually permed. I hugged my son. I was so happy to hear him say he loved my hair. Shortly after that, Shemar let his hair grow as he groomed it daily.

In fact, he began to embrace more black girls with natural hair. A blessing to see that I didn't realize was needed.

"I was wondering why you were about to cry. I love being black mama. I love your hair. I wish mine would grow like yours."

"Drink more water."

"Okay, this conversation is over." Shemar walked into his bedroom as I laughed out loud.

I stood in the mirror with the scissors as I thought back to the year 2008 when I cut my locs out of my hair after letting them grow for two years. I raised the scissors and cut the front of my hair off as I watched it fall into the sink and onto the floor. I stood there as my eyes filled with tears. I cut my hair and placed it in a plastic bag. I then grabbed the clippers and proceeded to cut the rest. About two weeks later, I sat at my computer and rubbed my head. The back felt strange and too smooth. I asked my son to take a picture of the back of my head as I had just broken my handheld mirror a week prior. The image blew my mind. It looked as if someone took a scalpel and not only cut my hair, but the skin underneath it was damaged, blotchy and inflamed just as my body was. I stared at the image in shock. The image was something I had never seen. I text Patrick the picture, and he texted me back.

"What the hell is going on?"

"Baby, just go back to the doctor. Somebody is fu***** up."

I cried. I was scared. In my twenty-three years of healthcare, I had seen a lot, but my head was something unusual.

"I already made an appointment."

"Okay. I will call you later. I'm on the dock and you know I can't be texting. I love you."

"I love you too."

I set my appointment to see the dermatologist for February eighth. I wanted answers. Something was eating me alive, and I refused to stop until I got answers. I changed my diet. I thought I was doing well. I had no flare ups or burning; only itching. But, apparently, something wasn't right on the inside. Even in the absence of the burning, my hair still fell out. What caused it? I thought. I wasn't ready to cut all of my hair off, so I borrowed a few of my sister's wigs, and bought a couple. I knew at some point; I would have to go bald.

"Hi, Mrs. Turner."

"Hi."

"How are you?"

I dropped my gown and exposed my naked body. Both doctors just stood there in awe. I could see the confusion in both of their faces.

"Mrs. Turner, I'm going to order some blood work on you. I need to check for any autoimmune disorders."

"That's fine. My hair has fallen out too. I took my wig off to expose my hair."

"I'm so sorry Mrs. Turner. I'm not sure what's going on. But let's get some blood work done and see what the results say."

The dermatologist ordered an antinuclear antibody, acute hepatitis; syphilis, tuberculosis, ssa and ssb antibody, cbc, comprehensive metabolic profile (CMP), and anti-dna double-stranded antibody. It doesn't make sense to elaborate on the different test as they were all negative as I thought they would be. But, you are welcome to google them. Thirty days before testing, I juiced and ate raw foods, so if any of those tests were positive, my diet changed it. But, was caused my hair to fall out? I didn't believe the alopecia garbage. Alopecia is the diagnosis doctors give when your hair falls out. But, what was the reason? Two weeks after my visit to the dermatologist, I went to see a naturopath physician. I told him everything I had done as didn't want to waste any more time. I told him about the fifteen pounds I released, my plant-based diet, the supplements I took, exercise and meditation. He was quite impressed as he stated. I even showed him an old image when I was heavier.

"I'm happy to know you have covered a lot of bases. Most patients come in and haven't done anything and want to make suggestions or request. What have other doctors said the issue was?

"I was diagnosed with Psoriasis and Pityriasis."

"That doesn't look like Psoriasis."

Dr. Nichols stared at my skin.

"I've never seen Psoriasis look this bad or follow this pattern."

"Me either. I had it when I was about twenty-five, and it lasted three weeks and was only in my chest area. There was no burning or skin peeling."

"So, what would you like to do today?"

"I want like to have a Leaky Gut test today."

"Okay, we can do that. What supplements are you taking?

"L-glutamine, licorice, enzyme digest, HCL, vitamin D...

"How many units?" Dr. Nichols interrupted me.

"Five thousand IU's of Vitamin D."

"Okay, that's good."

"What about a probiotic?"

"I'm taking a thirty billion capsule daily."

"Okay, good. You're taking the right supplement to heal the gut. So let's do a food sensitivity test."

"How many tubes of blood do you need?

"About ten. Dr. Nichols grabbed the tubes and needles out the drawer.

"What? You have got to be kidding me."

"I am." Dr. Nichols laughed.

I laughed out loud. *Thank God.* I thought.

"I only need one tube of blood."

"Thank God. How long before the test results come back."

"It could be three weeks or more. The test is performed on the East coast as Illinois does not do the food sensitivities test. They only do food allergies, and there is a huge difference. Also, the results come through the mail."

"Okay, will you call me or do I need to call you."

"I will call you, and we can set up your next appointment after the test results arrive."

"Okay. Thank you."

That test cost me four hundred and eighty dollars as Dr. Nichols didn't take insurance as no naturopath does. They also do not prescribe pills. I felt a sense of relief as I was finally getting somewhere. I left the doctor's office feeling sure and happy. Pat felt a sense of relief as well. We thought we were well on our way to healing. As much as I suffered, Pat did as well.

One week after my visit with Dr. Nichols, I suffered again. My body burned and the itch was unbearable. I was sure something was in my blood or underneath my skin. I went to ER at Metro South Medical Center (MSMC).

"Hi Mrs. Turner, I'm Dr. Allen. My nurse told me about your skin condition. How can we help you?"

"In the past, doctor's diagnosed me with Psoriasis, and this is nothing like before."

"So you've had Psoriasis in the past? Are you able to sit down?

"My skin hurts, and yes I have."

"Okay, well if the University of Chicago diagnosed you, I highly doubt that there is anything we can do?

The thing that pissed me off about this doctor was that he stood about six feet away from me and asked questions. In his mind, I was contagious. He never asked me any other questions as he never offered me anything for pain. I wanted to cuss that man out. He just walked out the room, and I cried. I worked for MSMC for five years, and one thing I know to be true is many of the ER nurses, and doctors assume most patients who seek pain relief seek morphine. I beg to differ. I would've been happy with the right diagnosis. I would've been glad if Dr. Allen had expressed his concern or interest.

I laid in that bed in so much pain. My skin felt like it ripped off my body. I cried until my nostrils filled with mucus.

"Hi, Mrs. Turner."

"Hi." I wiped my face and noticed a new doctor came in the room.

"I'm Dr Lilly. What's going on?

"There is something in my blood. If I'm not itching, or burning from the inside, my skin is peeling and inflamed. I cried as I bent over on the ER bed.

"What do you mean something is in your blood?"

"I can feel something moving around in me, like under my skin. Then it burns from the inside. I can't sleep at all. Please help me."

"Mrs. Turner there is nothing is your blood."

Dr. Lilly responded with conviction, but I wasn't convinced. If it wasn't in my blood, then what caused me to burn from the inside? Why did it feel like something crawled underneath my skin? Eventually, that doctor left, and another doctor came in. She was young, black and pretty, fair skinned, slim build and the only one who genuinely expressed interest and concern.

"Hi Mrs. Turner, I'm Dr. Shawn; I've talked to the other doctors so let me take a look at your skin."

I wanted to hear anything other than Psoriasis and Pityriasis, and I did. After carefully examining my body and asking several questions. The doctor stated I had Lichen Planus.

"What's Lichen Planus?"

"It's an inflammation of the skin caused by fungus. You need to see another doctor who can prescribe you the proper medicine. You will need to have your liver monitored as you will have to take antifungals."

"Can you prescribe it for me?"

"No. I cannot. But, I can set you up with a doctor for a follow-up appointment. So, let me get your discharge papers ready."

"Okay. Thank you. Finally, I was happy to hear something different as I thought I was going to get the proper medicine."

While Dr. Shawn worked on my discharge papers, I looked up Lichen Planus on google. The images were exactly like mine, and in fact, the rash was identical. I noticed a picture of the inside of someone's mouth, and there were white lines and white spots around the gum area and inner cheek. I had the same thing in my mouth. *Finally, a diagnosis that made sense.* I thought. I saw the first doctor in the hallway and approached him.

"Doctor, can I chat with you for a minute?"

"Sure."

"Dr. Shawn said my skin condition is Lichen Planus, a fungal infection or inflammation of the skin."

"Oh wow, I didn't even think of that. I apologize for not doing a deeper examination. I'm happy you feel better. I've never seen anything like that, so I wasn't sure. But, I should've asked more questions."

"Thanks for apologizing. I feel a lot better now."

"So, what exactly are you going to do now?"

"Well, I have to see another doctor outside of Metro. So Dr. Shawn is writing a referral for me to see another doctor. She said I would need to be on antifungal medicine and to have my liver monitored."

"Okay, well good luck to you."

"Thank you."

It's good to see that doctor had a heart and not just some asshole who thought I was contagious. I thought.

"Okay Kelley, I have your discharge papers. Here is a list of doctors you can choose from."

"Doctor, I looked up Lichen Planus on google, and there are images of the skin rashes that look just like mine and following the same patterns on my skin. My hair has fallen out as well."

"Lichen Planus will do that."

"Where does it come from?"

"Lichen Planus is one of those conditions that we don't have an answer for."

"Okay, well at least I know now what it is."

"In the meantime, here is some Tylenol to help you with the pain."

"Thanks doctor."

Pat and I left the hospital feeling somewhat relieved. The next morning I made an appointment with one of the doctors from the list Dr. Shawn gave me. This doctor was from Nigeria and did the typical as he was clueless about Lichen Planus. Although he did offer me a detox soup, he had no method of healing my body. I allowed him to draw blood, but I never went back for the test results. I lost faith in doctors. I began to lose respect for the entire healthcare industry. I realized the term "practicing" was what it was, practicing medicine. As in, I (doctors) am practicing medicine; you are a guinea pig and if I get it right, very good and if not, sue me. I mean, what is the purpose of malpractice insurance. Why do doctors need protection? Doctor's need protection because they have no idea of what healing means or entails.

I spent twenty-three years in the healthcare industry, and the best part of my job was when I spent time with the patients, talking to and comforting them. I loved working with patients and bringing a smile to their faces or cracking a joke to brighten their day. I loved the direct connection, not drawing blood or testing their blood or body fluids for dis-ease. It was too impersonal, and after watching the doctors at the University of Chicago Hospital kill patients and sweep it under the carpet or cause permanent damage to others, I became sickened by the lack of love for humans and the desire to protect a system. I became desensitized to death as I watched so much of it. In the beginning, it was depressing, but after a while, I became numb. Patients have died in my arms while treating them or assisting the doctors. Four years of death, mistakes, malpractice, and lies was enough for me. I decided to get my degree in medical technology and work in the back scene or the laboratory. In the lab, I didn't see the patient die, but based on their results; I could tell if they were dying or already dead. Just as watching my skin cells die, I had enough of watching patients die.

One week after seeing Dr. Nichols, I was on fire and inflamed again. My legs were very red and warm. I called Dr. Nichols, and after explaining the situation to him, he advised me to take one week of steroids to calm my immune system. I did that, and the inflammation subsided. The steroids purpose is to "turn off" my body or immune system process. Since my immune system was naturally attacking something, my body was profoundly affected to a degree of severe crying and suffering. I was happy to get some relief. However, I know steroids do significant damage to the gut, so I never retook steroids. I never gave up on seeking out a remedy, so this time I went to see a Chinese doctor, Dr. Yung. I had nothing to lose and everything to gain. Dr. Yung took my pulse, examined my tongue and asked several questions. He examined my legs and stomach and said toxic, toxic, very bad toxicity. He got up from his chair and walked over to his shelves and grabbed four bottles of herbs. Two were called Blood Stasis and the other two named Skin Wind. I took eighteen pills a day or six tablets three times a day from each bottle. They were tiny and easy to swallow.

I had enough pills for twenty-two days. I recall taking a shower, and after washing my feet, I noticed they were lighter than usual. I have always had a callus on my heels. One was thicker than the other, however, on this day, both of the calluses were gone. I also noticed the hyperpigmentation surrounded by lighter areas.

"Patrick!!!! I yelled, look, my callus disappeared, and my skin is clearing. My heels are light skinned."
WOW!!! I cried. *Finally, something works*. I thought.
"Look at my skin. Yasssssssssss!!! Thank you, Universe."
"Wow. Wow. Alright. You better keep taking those herbs."
"I am. One is for my blood, and the other is for my skin. I wonder what's in my blood. Dr. Yung said toxic several times. I wonder what it could be."
"Well baby, at least you found a doctor who knows what the hell he's talking about."
"Tell me about it."
"This is good. This is very good. I have to look these herbs up again."

Toxic; what's in my body? Leaky gut; how do they correlate? What's leaking into my bloodstream? Toxins, but what toxins? It is gluten, wheat, lectin, GMO's, what is it? I thought.

I continued to take the herbs from Dr. Yung as I made one more doctor's appointment at U of C. I wanted to see if a new doctor could confirm the Lichen Planus diagnosis. Although at this time, I knew the issue was more in-depth than my skin, I still wanted to hear what the dermatologist had to say about the Lichen Planus diagnosis. Almost a month passed before I received my food sensitivity test results. In my early twenties, doctors at the University of Chicago hospital diagnosed me with wheat corn, shellfish, ash tree and dust allergens. Well, according to the IgG Elisa 184 food panel test, it was the total opposite. I was sensitive to clam, cod, mussel, scallop and squid, malt, asparagus, mushrooms, radish, okra, and spinach. The list goes on as black-eyed peas, blackberries, cherries, fig, grapes and pineapples, almonds, cashew, macadamia, pine nuts, and sesame were all on the list.

Wheat and gluten were negative for sensitivity. So what exactly were the doctors at U of C talking about when they diagnosed me with wheat allergies? For whatever reason, I continued to see doctors at the U of C knowing they made many mistakes. I didn't know what else to do. I continued to research, ask questions, read, alter my diet, but I still missed something.

I certainly missed wearing clothing, but at this time, my skin had healed enough for apparel not to bother me. I was happy about that. I was still in a lot of emotional pain and confused about what caused such damage to my skin. I refused to give up, just as I refused to give up when I was confined to that bedroom for three years and drugged and raped. I have experienced some horrible things in my life and not only survived, but I thrived. This experience was no different. I knew something phenomenal was coming as without darkness; there can be no light. I was not only prepared; I was ready to receive whatever the Universe had for me and embraced whatever I created. It was just a matter of time before I found what I sought. Seek, and you shall find. Well, I did not stop until I discovered the truth. But, I made one last trip to U of C hospital.

Light Therapy

On March 7th, 2017, I saw Dr. Hea. Before my appointment, I called the risk management team at U of C to report the misdiagnosis on behalf of Dr. Dehti. I explained to the department manager, Sharon, how Dr. Dehti misdiagnosed me with Psoriasis and Pityriasis Rosacea. I also shared how I wanted to see another doctor there, but not her. Sharon set me up with one of their more experienced dermatologists, and I scheduled the appointment. I didn't know what to expect, but I prepared myself.

A nurse entered the room and asked the typical questions.
On a scale of one to ten, what is your pain level? Are you still taking the listed prescribed medicines? Do you need any refills? Do you have a cough or a sneeze? Do you understand our speak up program? Do you mind undressing and putting on this robe?

The same questions, plus a few more and I wasn't interested in talking to her as I wanted to talk to the doctor. The nurse finally left, and Dr. Napo walked in.
Dr. Napo was white, about five feet ten inches, handsome, brown hair and very kind.
"Hi there Mrs. Turner, how are you?"
Pat wasn't with me this day as he wasn't able to take off work. Even with the FMLA, we needed the money as he had already missed many days.
I immediately cried and dropped my robe. "This is how I'm doing. One of the doctors diagnosed me with Psoriasis, and she was wrong. What is this on my body?"
Dr. Napo moved in closer to me and examined my body.
"This is not Psoriasis; this is Lichen Planus."
"That is what the ER doctor at Metro South said."
"Really?"
"Yes."
"Great, well let me get the attending physician to confirm. But, will it be okay if we did a biopsy to diagnose properly. I'm one

hundred percent certain it is Lichen Planus, but I know you had some issues before, so we want to be sure."

"That is fine."

"Okay, let me gey the attending."

Dr. Napo left for about five minutes and returned with this tall, white, older doctor. I can tell he had practiced medicine for over twenty years.

"Hi Mrs. Turner, I'm doctor Hea, I'm sorry about the trouble you had with the previous doctors, but, looking at you now, I'm one hundred percent certain you have Lichen Planus. Dr. Napo mentioned a biopsy to me, and that is the diagnostic procedure we use to confirm the diagnosis. You have experienced so much pain already so I won't bother to cause you anymore. I've been a doctor for over twenty years as I have made numerous Lichen Planus diagnosis. So, if you trust me, I can confirm the diagnosis without a biopsy. You don't need to feel any more pain."

"That is fine and thank you. I don't want any more pain. Thank you, doctor." I cried.

Dr. Hea left the room. I cried out of relief that finally, we had something sound. But there was still more to this experience. Dr. Napo was very compassionate. He even hugged me. He was one of the kindest and most compassionate doctors that's ever treated me at U of C hospital.

"Kelley, do you mind if I have a few students come in and take a few images. I have never seen Lichen Planus at this level."

"Sure, why not. An image can't hurt." We laughed.

Two white, young women came in and took images. I stood their nude, raised my arms over my head, spun around and allowed them to take pictures of my body that would be used later as a teaching tool. I was okay with that. Dr. Napo came back in the room.

"Kelley, are you familiar with light therapy?"

"I have heard of it through a few people who have received it."
"Light therapy will help lighten up the dark spots on your body."

"Well, I guess it won't hurt to try."

I don't want any of this traditional medicine bullshit. I want freedom from this healthcare system and these practicing doctors. I thought.

I recalled a Facebook friend told me she had used Light Therapy and it worked everywhere but in her scalp. That didn't convince me to try it, but, after trying everything else, why not.

"Okay, excellent Kelley. Here is the order for the Light Therapy and a stronger steroid. You will have the therapy twice a week for ten weeks starting tomorrow. When you schedule it, make sure the appointments are at least a day apart."

Dr. Napo left the room, and I gathered my belongings and left the room. He prescribed a different steroid, but I didn't use it. I decided I was done with pharmaceutical drugs as I knew one day I would stop taking the Levothyroxine for my thyroid. I visited Dr. Yung in Chinatown and purchased my herbs. I finally found something that worked so I wasn't going to stop taking the herbs.

My body didn't burn as much as it did in the beginning. I maintained a diet with vegetables, juices and a plant-based diet. I rarely had meat, and if I did, it was only chicken. The light treatment consisted of me standing upright in a tanning booth as to me that is what it was. After about nine or ten treatments, I noticed blisters on my skin on top of the rashes on my outer thigh and on my left ankle.

I sent Dr. Napo a message, and he responded in this manner.
Message
From: Dr. L Napo
Sent: 4/14/2017 10:35 AM CDT
To: Kelley Porter-Turner
Subject: RE: Follow up Question

Hello Ms. Porter-Turner,
Sorry to hear you had some blistering. We want to take a week break from the light therapy and put you on another steroid taper. Same instructions as before, we will do 40mg day one, 30 mg day two, 20 mg day three, 10 mg day four, and 5 mg day five. Then restart the light therapy. I sent the medication to your pharmacy. Thank you for updating us! Via my chart.

Every damn solution in healthcare is a pill. I did not use those steroids. Steroids are known for destroying the lining of the intestines so if I have gut issues, why the hell would I want to add fuel to the fire. Later that day, I responded to Dr. Napo.

Dr. Napo,
I have been seeing a holistic, integrative physician along with you all and my integrative doctor diagnosed me with Leaky Gut. I had a 184 (ELISA) food sensitivity test done, and the results were positive for numerous food and spice sensitivities; symptoms of Leaky Gut. When I was seventeen, doctors at Jackson park hospital diagnosed me with a peptic ulcer. I assumed it was from taking the Ibuprofen for an extended time as I know steroids destroy the intestinal lining. I understand you all treat the symptoms of the underlying disease as that is what Western medicine has done since conception. However, the steroids will only suppress my immune system as we hope the inflammatory response goes away. That is not the case. I have intestinal permeability, and it needs treatment. I avoid all the foods I'm sensitive too, but the food particles, molecules, and undigested food leaks into my bloodstream and cause my body to become inflamed.

So, as you know I am suffering from Lichens Planus (symptom), but the underlying disease is Leaky Gut. Leaky Gut or digestive issues are also the reason doctors diagnosed me with Hypothyroidism. The gluten molecule mimics or looks like my thyroid molecule, so when the gluten or lectin destroyed the walls of my intestinal lining and leaked into my bloodstream, my body went into defense mode or autoimmune and attacked my thyroid. This is the same case now, but my skin is being attacked. I do not want to suffer any longer. I am tired of my body burning, itching and so forth. I cannot focus on school, work, and my marriage is rocky as I am not myself emotionally, mentally or physically, Please, can we look at an alternative method of treatment. Is there a surgery that involves placing a mesh into my stomach or intestines to stop the leaking?

I am tired of burning as some days my clothing hurts. I don't want to eat anything. I cannot take this any longer. Please step outside of traditional medicine and treat my whole body. I know you all are capable. Please help me and heal the Leaky Gut. You are probably wondering how I know these things. I have over 20 years of experience working as a Medical Technologist, and today I am a Holistic Life Coach. My whole body needs treatment and if you do not believe you can heal me, then let stop right here.

Thank you,
Kelley P. Turner

Response
Hello Ms. Porter-Turner,

I want to first start off by saying I respect your decision and your way of life. I also wanted to give you a little more background on Lichen Planus. Lichen Planus is an inflammatory disorder in which your immune system attacks its cells. We, the medical community, do not know exactly how this condition arises or what causes it. We know that it is, as I have said above, an inflammatory reaction in which your body's defensive cells will attack specific cells within the skin, causing a rash that we see from the outside. This condition has been linked with specific infectious processes like Hepatitis C (for which you are negative) and associated with trauma. I went through all the literature, and I could not find a single association of Lichen Planus and leaky gut. I also wanted to let you know, though I respect your integrative physician's opinion, that the vast majority of leaky gut cases were due to surgical removal of part of the gastrointestinal tract, and not from peptic ulcer disease. I would just be careful and make sure you ask them to show you scientific proof as to why you have leaky gut, I am sure they probably have it as this seems to be their area of expertise, but I would have them show it to you none the less. Back to the Lichen Planus, because we know that it is an inflammatory disease, we use an anti-inflammatory measure to treat it, such as the steroids and the phototherapy. We are not addressing your symptoms; we are treating the condition. Lichen Planus has been studied for many years, and we know that the majority of cases do respond to the treatments that we discussed, with few, unfortunately, becoming unresponsive, which we hope is not your case. We can only give you the medical opinion on what has been scientifically studied. Many holistic practices are good in theory, but end up not being more effective than a sugar pill. Meaning the body probably resolved whatever the condition was on its own, and thus the holistic intervention did not hold up to the scientific method.

Those that do pass the scientific method eventually work their way into "western" medicine. Which brings me to my next point. The majority of Lichen Planus cases resolve entirely on their own within two years' time without any intervention at all. I leave it to you. As I said, I completely respect your viewpoint and your way of life, and your integrative physician's opinion, and if you would like to stop treatment with us and work solely with them, I will respect that as well. The orders are placed for your steroid taper and your light therapy, it is up to you if you choose to use them.

Have a happy Easter,

Great Rising Dr
Thank you for responding. Please read the article below. And the doctor I'm working with is a Medical Doctor who left the hospitals to focus on integrative or functional medicine. He treats the whole person and not symptoms. I will continue the light therapy, but steroids destroy the digestive tract as well so I won't take them. I will call the phototherapy office on Monday and let them know I have to skip a week from the therapy. I've been using natural blood cleansers (herbs) and avoiding the foods my body is sensitive too. I have a question for you. You said Lichens Planus is an inflammatory response to something, but you are unsure of what; my question is, wouldn't you be curious to know what's causing any beautiful and magnificent body to attack itself. When we have our blood drawn we draw from the venous blood because it is "dirty" blood. How does blood get dirty? Foods, GMO's, lectin, gluten and other dangerous products destroy our digestive system. The father of medicine, Hippocrates said 2000

years ago that 80% of dis-ease starts in the gut. If we heal our guts, we heal our whole bodies.

I thank you for using what you've been taught to help heal me, and I respect you and the healthcare industry. But, at some point doctors have to be re-educated on the body, nutrition, and healing. Please review the article and I look forward to seeing you again as you were very kind to me. You treated me as a person and not just a patient. Thank you, and I would say Happy Easter, but I don't celebrate it.

I sent the link below for Dr. Napo to read.
http://www.skinsensibility.com/leaky-gut-syndrome-and-why-it-could-be-important-to-your-skin/

After the dialogue with Dr. Napolitano, I decided to ditch light therapy and continue taking the Chinese herbs. I avoided sugar, flour, coffee, dairy, bad carbs, starchy foods and meat as well and any other inflammatory or mucus-producing food. The flares ups ended, and I felt better about healing.

Spring 2017
I felt some discomfort within my mind as I worried about the warm weather and wearing clothing that exposed my body. I dealt with the emotions surrounding the skin issues, but I had not dealt with the fear surrounding my body. At this time, black, raised rashes covered seventy percent of my body. You could not see my tattoos at all. Black, dark, raised outbreaks were all over my hamstrings, thighs, side and between my legs, calves, and the front of my calves, stomach, arms, and feet. So many days, I thought my skin was disgusting. I thought I was disgusting. I even embraced the diagnosis as Lichen Planus as in the video I shared, clearly stated my Lichen Planus. I had to change my thoughts, my words and beliefs. I thought about what life would be like walking around in the summer. What people would say and how they would start. Even when the flares ups, itching and burning subsided, I had another issue to deal with; I had to learn

to truly love and accept myself in the midst of feeling ugly, disgusting and unattractive.

But, how was I to help anyone in the midst of misery? Well, in the middle of my pain, sharing and talking about it, helped me heal internally. On April 15th, 2017, I went live on FB as my husband scanned my entire body. Right before I shared that video, I was afraid and very nervous. I was scared of what people would think of me, how they would perceive me and what people would say. I asked Patrick what he thought of the idea of sharing my skin publicly.

"Pat I'm going to expose my body live on FB for the world to see. I think exposing myself will help me remove the shame and help others do the same."

"Well, if that's what you want to do, I'm with you."

"I'm scared."

"Don't be baby; this is what you do. You've been using your life to help others for a long time, and this is no different. You will be fine. Just let me know when you are ready for me to video you."

"Should I just wear my bra or put a shirt on and then raise the shirt up?"

"I think you should just wear the bra and some shorts."

"Okay. I will do that."

Moments later, I picked my phone up and pressed live and wrote; Exposing my body. Lichens Planus. Removing the shame & helping you do the same. After that, I pushed go live. The video was twelve minutes and eighteen seconds, and directly afterward, Pat took me out to have lunch.

That video went viral. To this current day, the video I shared has been over 320,000 and shared over 7,800 times, and when Vashty Victor from Liberia shared it, the views quadrupled to over 1.8 million views and 25,000 shares.

Video link
https://www.facebook.com/KelleyPorterT/videos/4433332493
35799

I received hundreds, of messages from people across the world. People from every continent except Antarctica reached out to thank me, and express their experiences with what doctors diagnosed as skin disorders. Every message sent, represented love, inspiration, hope, sadness and joy. People praised my transparency and ability to show the world what society deemed as ugly yet, I stood firm in it and used my pain to not only empower others but empower and heal myself. So many people shared their skin disorders and depression with me. I was completely amazed. In fact, in May of 2017 a journalist from Cameroon, Afrika interviewed me. I realized at that moment; my experience was a lot larger than me and in fact, it wasn't even about me.

That was the first day I went outside to expose my body. The back of my shirt was open, so people were able to see my back, arms, and legs. I felt comfortable when I was with Patrick. I felt protected by him as being outside with him made thing a lot easier than being alone. I got plenty of stares and still to do this day, I do. And that is okay. I understand people would instead hide than show their true self. But, I refuse to allow shame to suffocate me. I refuse to live my life worrying about what people think of me as it is none of my business. I am not my skin as my skin does not define me. Facebook live was the best decision I could have ever made as it catapulted my emotional and mental healing. Today, I see my hyperpigmentation as beauty marks. More importantly, my skin is beautiful with two shades of brown.

About a week after sharing that video, I received an invite to an Entrepreneur forum. I do not attend networking events; however, my spirit made sure I participated in this one. The young lady who invited me was someone I met about five years ago, and we reconnected on FB. Kara Scott posted an invite to an

Entrepreneur Forum, and I delightfully accepted the invite without hesitation. On that day, I met James Dentley, Kara's husband, as he offered me an $8,000 scholarship to attend their professional speaker's school, Network Business Building Coaching (NBC University). I was in awe and indeed happy to accept. On April 25th, I drove to Matteson, Illinois to attend my first day of professional speaker's school. The entire experience was terrific. Being trained by millionaires was fantastic as well as learning the information I did. I indeed use all that I have learned today. My gratitude still rings high for James and Kara. I love them. But, the most critical moment during those six, twelve hour days was meeting Marc Haygood. Marc Haygood played a significant role in my life as he is the reason my spirit led me to say yes when Kara invited me to her entrepreneur forum. Again, I never attend entrepreneur or network events.

Everything that happened after that moment and before was all in divine order. I was supposed to say yes as saying yes to Kara was saying yes to all the information and knowledge I sought after. If Kara had not invited me on that day, I would probably still flare up, burn, itch and be nowhere near as healed as I am today. Kara, Marc, and James changed my life, and I am so grateful the Universe sent me exactly who I needed.

The information I received shocked me and was right on point as I embraced it and moved forward in healing. What I found was unbelievable, unimaginable and proof that all disease starts in the gut. What's more, millions, maybe billions of us are walking host for intestinal worms and an overgrowth of yeast.

Turpentine and Castor Oil

On the elevator with two other students, we exited as we came to the first floor of the 600 Office Building in Matteson, Illinois.

"Hey, what's your name?"

"My name is Marc."

"I'm Kelley; we haven't sat together yet. Let's sit and work together tomorrow. I mean that's what's we're supposed to do, right? Move around and sit with other students."

"Did they say that?"

"Yeah, James said it today as well."

"Okay."

"Well, alright." Marc smiled, and we both walked toward the exit door."

"Have a good night and see you tomorrow."

"You too Kelley."

Marc and I said our goodbyes and the next day we forgot to sit together. We laughed about, but had some dialogue about his detox program. Marc was very kind and easy to talk too. I took an immediate liking to him. His energy was very calm and collected. After practicing our presentations together, I heard a lot about Marc's detox program, and by day three, Marc shared with me something that I never even thought. But, I sought out information, and as I know, if you seek you will find. The Universe aligned me with every step before the day Marc shared with the truth about my body.

Since August of 2016, I researched, saw numerous doctors, took herbs, and did light therapy, acupuncture, read books and so much more. I diligently looked for answers as I asked the Universe to help me. By day three Marc shared with me the information I sought after.

"Kelley, I believe you have parasites."

"Really."

"Yeah."

"My wife, or ex-wife, had them too and her skin was messed up. Those things were trying to come through her skin."

"Really?" I crossed my arms and looked into Marc's eyes.

"Try this. Buy some turpentine and castor oil and take that for a couple of days. In fact, google Jennifer Daniels; she has the entire protocol of getting rid of parasites with turpentine. Or just go on you tube and watch the stories about turpentine and removing parasites."

"I'm working with this guy right now. Well, I made an appointment to have the biometric screening done."

"What's his name?"

"Eric. Eric Prince."

"I know him."

"For real? Cool. Well, I'm going to have this test done, and I will keep you posted."

"Alright, but yeah, go on YouTube and look up Dr. Jennifer Daniels too."

"Okay, thanks, Marc."

Our break ended, and it was time for us to get back to work. I was excited to hear what Marc told me. I wasn't excited about the parasites, but I was delighted to hear something that might be the answer to my healing crisis. The moment I got home, I googled Dr. Jennifer Daniels and listened to her interview about healing dis-ease with turpentine and castor oil. I was shocked to hear that the same turpentine the FDA told us was dangerous, is the exact turpentine our ancestors used to heal the slave masters. In fact, there was a skull head and a big X on the bottle. Pure Gum Spirits of Turpentine to worms is like raid to roaches and yeast.. According to Dr. Daniels, the moment the turpentine touches your tongue, the worms and yeast immediately runs for the exit or your anus. However, a blocked colon will trigger them to run upwards towards your lungs. That might sound a bit over the top, but, it is true as I experienced the exact thing Dr. Daniels shared. I decided to wait before I tried the turpentine as I wanted to do the biometric screening to determine what organs if any, were in a critical state. After doing the test, I learned my digestive system was in the worse state as my liver was considered slightly fatty.

After I completed that test, I decided to go ahead and purchase the turpentine and castor oil. On May 3rd, 2017, I bought the Pure Gum Spirits of Turpentine only to receive a package that read 100% Pure Essential Oil of Pine Tree. I called the merchant and was told, 100% Pure Gum Spirits of Turpentine was exactly what was in the bottle. I wasn't convinced, so I ordered one from Diamond G products on May 8th, 2017.

While waiting for my new bottle of turpentine, I received a message from the former merchant stating when turpentine ships to America; the bottle has to be packaged in that matter to be received in America. I was in complete disbelief. Why would America not want pure gum spirits of turpentine shipped to America? I didn't ask, but, it doesn't take a rocket scientist to figure out if the Europeans didn't bring our ancestor's healing remedies to America when they stole us from Africa, why would they allow others to sell it to us from other countries? Healthcare is a business and never created for healing purposes. If that were the case, why are so many people suffering from dis-ease and dying? There is undoubtedly a gap between the two and what I released from my body shed a lot of light on dis-ease and death in America.

I texted Eric Prince and told him I wanted to do the turpentine and castor oil first before trying any herbs. I also trusted the merchant and moved forward with the turpentine and castor oil. I read Dr. Daniel's protocol, but I didn't follow the complete instructions. A part of the instructions was to open the colon and give the parasites and yeast a way out. When Dr. Daniels said the parasites and yeast would seek an immediate way out and by any means necessary, she wasn't lying. Obviously, my colon was blocked as I felt the worms or yeast coming up through my throat. I gagged and choked. I called Marc the next day and explained the situation to him.

"Hey Marc."
"Hey, hey."

"So, I did the turpentine and castor oil and it felt like something tried to crawl up through my lungs. I choked and gagged."

"Oh yeah, you have to make sure your colon is open because they will try to exit any hole."

"Okay, so what do I do now?"

"I'm going to bring you some colon sweep. I will stop by tomorrow and don't use the turpentine until your colon is open. Have you ever heard of a coffee enema?"

"No, I have not."

"A coffee enema is just like the water and ACV except you're using organic coffee."

"Really, so I'm putting coffee in my ass."

"Yep." Marc laughed.

"You purchase some organic coffee and boil it the same way you would make your coffee. Let it cool off, filter it and then add it to the bag. Once you do the enema, you have to hold it in for fifteen minutes. And you have to lie on your right side. But, you have to make sure you can get the entire bag of water in you. If you cannot get the entire bag of water in you, then you will not get half the bag of coffee in you."

"Okay. I'm going to buy some coffee and do one tomorrow."

"The coffee enema detoxifies your liver immediately. Do it for seven days straight. But be sure to get the entire bag of water in you first. And you're going to feel high as ever." Marc laughed.

"Okay. I will text you when I get the coffee."

Over the next three days, I took the colon sweep and released regularly. I purchased organic coffee from Whole Foods and researched coffee enemas. Marc was right on the money. I needed to detox my liver and all other elimination channels or organs. By day four, I was ready to try the coffee enema.

Text message

Hey Marc, the coffee is boiling, and I'm about to do a coffee enema. But I'm doing the ACV first.

I used distilled water and filled the two-quart enema bag and added a tablespoon of apple cider vinegar (ACV) in it.

Text message

Marc, the entire bag went in. Yayyyyy. I'm flushing now. I'm going to take the turpentine and castor oil, and the coffee as soon as I finish flushing.

Marc: That's good. The colon sweep opened you up.

Me: Thank you so much as meeting you was all in divine order. I asked for you.

Marc: Thank you

Me: You're welcome. Ttyl (Talk to you later)

I flushed for about twenty minutes. The waste looked very old and like something from the sewage. After flushing, I took the turpentine and castor oil, and after that, I laid in the bathtub and inserted the tubing into my rectum. I released the clamp and immediately closed the clamp. The tubing was full of coffee.

I don't want any coffee ground in my ass. Let me release some of this sh** and the air and try again. I thought.

I released the air and coffee ground and laid back in the tub. Finally, all the coffee was in me. I got up and went into my bedroom and laid on my right side. I set the clock for fifteen minutes and played candy crush. Candy crush distracted me from focusing on the time. After about three minutes, the coffee surged towards my anus, and I had to squeeze my butt cheeks and breathe. That surge came at least four more times. But, I held that coffee in and after fifteen minutes, I got up and ran to the bathroom. I released a toilet full of pinworms. I was in complete shock. I took pictures of what looked like rice particles as I remembered what they looked like when I was 8 years old. They were smaller than an inch long and white. I was happy and felt energized; however, I knew there was more to come.

Dr. Daniels spoke of candida in her interview, so I went to Google and YouTube University again to see the appearance of yeast. By day five, I released a lot of yeast and took pictures of that as well. I was in complete disbelief. I wasn't convinced the pinworms or the amount of yeast I saw was the end of this experience. I continued to take the turpentine and castor oil, along with the coffee and ACV enemas. I did the coffee enemas for seven days as I did the ACV enema for a complete thirty days. Some days after the coffee and water enema, I felt drained and weak. I felt sick. I wasn't sure why, but I learned later. I also experienced hives, headaches, my body burned, but I did not have any new rashes. But that hot flash-like feeling came back as I felt nauseated. I called Marc and was amazed by the information he shared with me.

"Kelley, you're experiencing "Die-Off." Google it, die off is when the worms and yeast die."
"Okay, this is crazy. My body is burning like before."
"When you experience that, eat a big salad or do an enema."
"Okay. Thanks, Marc. I will keep you posted.

I googled 'Die Off' and was amazed at the information. Die-Off symptoms are synonymous to what doctors diagnose. According to the Candida Diet website, when large numbers of yeast and fungal cells are rapidly killed, a die-off (or Herxheimer reaction, healing crisis) occurs, and metabolic by-products release into the body. The amount of candida cells killed makes this very different from the regular cell elimination that forms part of the candida albicans lifecycle (Perfect Health, Ltd).

The Herxheimer Reaction is a short-term (from days to a few weeks) detoxification reaction in the body. As the body detoxifies, it is not uncommon to experience flu-like symptoms including a headache, joint and muscle pain, body aches, sore throat, general malaise, sweating, chills, nausea or other symptoms (unknown internet source).

The name Jarisch-Herxheimer is the official name given to the physical reactions from the release of toxins by the dying Candida because the two dermatologists who discovered the die-off reaction were Karl Herxheimer and Adolf Jarisch, (Brookwood 2013). How ironic is it that two dermatologists discovered this information as it makes me wonder if all dermatologists are aware of this die-off and refuse to treat the candida infestation. To treat the candida infestation means to heal the patient and therefore not receive another check.

When candida cells die, they release all the harmful substances that they contain, including (according to some sources) at least 79 different toxins. This long list of toxic substances includes ethanol, uric acid, and acetaldehyde (Perfect Health Ltd). Acetaldehyde, a known neurotoxin, has a whole host of detrimental effects on your health and wellbeing. It can impair your brain function and even kill brain cells. Your endocrine, immune and respiratory systems can all be affected, and it also damages the membranes of your red blood cells, reducing their ability to carry oxygen through the body. You can see how excess acetaldehyde can quickly contribute to non-specific symptoms like brain fog and fatigue. These harmful by-products also cause allergic reactions and inflammation that lead to an array of troublesome symptoms (Perfect Health Ltd, no year).

Die-Off symptoms are sometimes compared to those of a common cold or seasonal allergies but can be considerably different from person to person. The toxic by-products of candida tend to cause inflammation, which can lead to a stuffy nose, blocked sinuses and other allergy-like symptoms. Metabolites like the neurotoxin acetaldehyde can also cause symptoms like brain fog, headaches, fatigue, and nausea. Remember that these toxins are stressing your liver too, so having a sore abdomen (especially in the liver region) is also possible (Perfect Health Ltd, no year). I am grateful I never experienced pain on my right side or my abdomen.

The die-off reaction includes **fatigue, yeast infections, joint pain, brain fog, frequent colds, oral thrush, headaches, mood swings, dizziness, itching, acne, sinus congestion, bloating & gas.** Die off symptoms also includes **weight gain, urinary infections, food cravings, irritability, food sensitives, insomnia, abdominal pain and red, itchy eyes.** Lastly, Die Off symptoms include **rashes, Psoriasis/Eczema , and allergies**

(Perfect Health, Let me add Lichen Planus to the list. How interesting is that? Every condition listed is precisely what doctors diagnose thereby treating a symptom rather than your whole body. And I am almost sure some if not many of the traditional doctors are aware of this fact. You might wonder why some of the symptoms are in bold. The symptoms in bold are the ones I have personally experienced starting at the age of eight and up until now.

The following article was written by Dr. Jack Zoldan.
The candida syndrome, also known as the yeast syndrome, is a chronic disease caused by the over activity of the yeast; candida albicans. Candida is a common inhabitant of the non-sterile areas of the body, including the skin, the sinuses, the gastrointestinal tract, and the vagina. Optimally, it lives in peaceful co-existence with its host. Unfortunately, the yeast often gains dominance. Many temporary or long-term insults to the body [any of which I call "A Shock to the System"] can initiate a process which allows the overgrowth of candida. Once the organism becomes independently functioning, it leads to the many problems associated with the disease.

People who suffer from the candida syndrome often appear healthy. The results of medical testing are also normal. The frequently used blood test for candida antibody is not reliable for diagnosis. The candida syndrome is often associated with other chronic diseases, like chronic fatigue syndrome, lyme disease, fibromyalgia, IBS, headache, and depression, to name a few. A chronic illness makes the victim susceptible to the development of other problems. Thus, the candida syndrome often coexists with other diseases. The symptoms of these continuing obstacles overlap. Diagnosis and therapy must, therefore, be approached broad-mindedly.

The first stage in therapy of the candida syndrome, as in all chronic illness, is to recognize that there is a problem that needs addressing. One who suffers from the candida syndrome must be taken seriously. The next step is to begin the process of reclaiming health. People acquired the candida Syndrome because of an underlying health imbalance. I believe that an inadequately healthy lifestyle predisposed to the disease. Restoring such a lifestyle is the key to recovery. My experience in treating chronic conditions, including the candida syndrome, is that this is successful (Jack Zolden, 2005).

End Article.

On September 14 and 15, I had a massive die-off reaction. My lips swelled up, and there were hives all over my body, and no, I did not run to the doctor. I treated the reaction with hot lemon water and ACV. That was not the first time. I have experienced hives at least four times since I began healing my body without pharmaceutical drugs. Switching from processed foods to real foods starves the worms and yeast as starting an increased probiotic dosage causes death as well as the good bacterium dominates. In fact, I upped my probiotic to a 100 billion probiotic once a day. Since treating the candida and parasitic infestation, I experienced itching, mood swings, dizziness, nausea, headache, allergies, food sensitivities, cravings, and brain fog.

I recall back to when I was about thirty years young and had issues remembering as I lost my words in the middle of sentences. The doctors at U of C Hospital did a brain scan and found nothing. Now, I know why. According to Brookwood (2013), Acetaldehyde toxins are capable of killing brain cells, damaging the endocrine system and therefore causing an imbalance of hormones. Acetaldehyde also impairs the respiratory system, your immune system, and adrenal glands, as well as cause damage to red blood cells which carry oxygen to different organs and the throughout the body in general (Brookwood 2013). This helps you to understand why the die-off symptoms include such bothersome symptoms as brain fog, dizziness, and even the tired feeling; all because your body is not receiving an adequate supply of oxygen due to the aldehydes release by the dying candida (Brookwood 2013). Doctors diagnosed me with hypothyroidism in 2014. I wonder why. The thyroid is within the endocrine system and responsible for metabolism, growth, and maturation of the human body. The thyroid also helps to regulate body functions by releasing hormones into the bloodstream. Imagine that. Imagine how the toxins released by candida die off caused a lack of oxygen to all organs resulting in thyroid imbalance.

Today, I am happy to say; my thyroid is back to regular production. Doctors are quick to blame disease on old age and hereditary. Every dis-ease I experienced was directly related to yeast and worms die off. I no longer take any medicine. What's more, the some of the foods I was diagnosed as sensitive to are foods that starve yeast and worms eliciting a "die off," resulting in toxins released into my bloodstream. Spinach, asparagus, radish, okra cherries, grapes, and pineapples are all alkaline foods so how was my body sensitive to these healthy foods? How? The only conclusion I came up with was these alkaline foods starved the yeast and worms causing a die off, and at that point, my body reacted to the toxins released into my bloodstream. I am not sure about the others, but today, I can eat whatever I choose, I just eat to live and not die anymore.

Parasite die-off is very similar to candida die off as the symptoms are fever, muscle aches, chills, headaches, skin rashes, excess mucus production, brain fog and increased gastrointestinal problems such as constipation and diarrhea. Interestingly enough, I experienced all of those symptoms before this current healing crisis. I have images of worms wrapped up in excess mucus like a spider web holding a fly.

How many people around the world are suffering from yeast and worm infestations? The people we call the government and doctors are quick to say parasites are only found in countries like Mexico, Africa, or third world countries. I beg to differ. Millions of Americans are suffering from parasitic infestations and have no idea as doctors are either lying and or ignorant to the facts.

After researching die off, I made sure to do an enema whenever my body presented symptoms and before the mixed teaspoon of turpentine and teaspoon of castor oil, (T&C) I also made sure to drink at least half of my body weight in purified or spring water. I used distilled water and a tablespoon of ACV for the enemas. On days I didn't take the T & C, I exercised using YouTube videos. I wanted to keep moving and assist the peristalsis or intestinal muscle movement. I was happy to be on the right track. I took the T& C three days a week and exercised four days a week. I must say, those thirty days were mentally and physically draining. I was tired all the time, but life had to go on. I mustered up the energy I had in me and flew to Texas with Patrick and Shemar for Pat Jr's high school graduation. I didn't want to go as I knew drinking was involved, processed foods as well as meat. I tried to avoid anything that I was powerless to at that moment. What's more, I wanted to stay home as I didn't feel comfortable doing enemas and pooping in someone else's house. My focus was to heal my body and create optimal health.

I awoke early in the morning the day of Pat Jr's graduation. I did an enema and in the toilet was a pinworm. I wanted to see more than those little critters. I knew there was something more than the yeast and pinworms. Every day in Texas except the last day was drinking and partying as I created a party for the yeast and worms. I felt them moving around in me. This day took me back to the very first day I felt something moving restlessly inside of me. It was the parasites and yeast. It all made sense to me. On May 27th, we flew home. I suffered on that airplane. I scratched and itched like a dog.

I felt them moving from my feet to my head, neck, arms, and legs. I rubbed my head, squirmed in the seat, rubbed my legs and for at least an hour of that three-hour flight, my body was a playground. I was miserable. I wanted to cry, and in fact, I did, for a second. But it didn't make sense to feel sorry for myself; I did it. I fed those little critters, as I knew what the outcome was. So I sucked up it, took some deep breaths and relaxed my mind. I ignored them the rest of the flight and fell asleep. I awoke about twenty minutes before landing.

I'm fuc**** these things up when I get home. I cannot wait until we get off this plane. I thought. We arrived at O'Hare airport at about eleven thirty and didn't get home until well after midnight. Sunday morning, I immediately took the turpentine and castor oil, but the creepy crawly didn't subside until about a week later.

On May 28th, I finally released a six-inch worm and damn near passed out in the bathroom.

"Patrick, look at this sh**. A real fuc**** worm! Un-damn-believable."

There it was on the tissue paper.

"I feel like throwing up. I can't believe this isht came out of me. My goodness; I wonder how much more are inside of me. This is the shit I feel crawling around in me."

"Wow. Wow. That came out of you."

"Yes, hard to believe. Well, this is the damn proof right here. All that burning, itching, skin peeling and misery is because of the yeast and these damn worms dying and releasing toxins into my bloodstream. Well, guess what, I'm not going to stop until I get these fuc*** out of me. Un- fuc*** real."

I stared at that worm for about five minutes before I flushed it down the toilet. I was in disbelief. I sent the image to Marc via text, and he responded, yep, I told you. I was thirsty to see what else would come from my rectum. Daily, I used a fork, spoon, spatula, stick or anything else to dig in the bottom of the toilet to see what came out of me. I checked the toilet every single day and my goodness that worm was nothing compared to what was to come. I was livid but excited at the same time. I wanted those little niglets out of me. I was on a mission to conquer those aliens and heal my body. I didn't release another worm until towards the end of the thirty days. However, almost every day, I released yeast and pinworms.

I remember my mother using turpentine and castor oil when we were sick. The main thing I remember is that they were both nasty. Our ancestors used turpentine for healing their children, families and slave masters. According to Dr. Daniels, American slaves had a secret remedy that kept them free of diseases: a teaspoon of turpentine mixed with a teaspoon of white sugar, taken for short periods several times each year. The MSDS for Diggers Pure Gum Turpentine states: "Ingestion can cause nausea, vomiting and bladder irritation. Aspiration into lungs, when swallowed or vomited, may cause chemical pneumonitis which can be fatal" (Last, no year). Well, I am here, alive and well to tell you that when used correctly healing occurs, not dis-ease or death. According to Dr. Daniels, the maximum dose is one teaspoon if you weight between forty and two hundred forty pounds and enough to wreak havoc on worms and yeast.

My problem was not being one hundred percent sure of what to eat and what not to eat. I followed a lot of what Dr. Axe shared on what to eat when treating Candida and unfortunately I did not read all of what Dr. Jennifer Daniels authored. That was my first mistake. Dr. Daniels has coached clients to heal naturally since 1985, and I should've used her complete program in the beginning. If you recall, the yeast and parasites tried to come through my lungs as my colon wasn't clear. I eventually had to do the turpentine and castor oil again. I felt some relief, but not exactly what I needed. I released a lot of yeast and I mean a lot of it, and just as many pinworms. However, if you watched the video of my skin that was enough for me to know there was a whole lot more going on in my body. Seventy percent of my skin was damaged, burned and peeled as if some dangerous chemical spilled into my bloodstream. I believe if I had the perfect diet for my candida cleanse, the turpentine would have worked well. So, what did I do that didn't align with my healing? My diet was obviously not aligned with healing. I still ate chicken, almonds, cashew, and a few other foods that fed the yeast and worms. What's more, there had to have been a lot of waste inside my colon, and that is a breeding ground for parasites. My next step was to detox my body and flush my colon as I have lived a slow death long enough.

Marc's detox program was exactly what I needed before the turpentine and castor oil. However, trial and error are also what I needed to fully understand what it took to heal my body naturally.

From this day forward, there are a few products that will always take up space in my home. Those products are turpentine, castor oil, an enema bag, probiotics, apple cider vinegar, essential oils, shea butter, lemons, cayenne pepper, coconut and olive oil, cinnamon, turmeric, basil, and a few others. I am one hundred percent for natural healing. Although the process takes a lot longer than drugs do, I think it is highly fascinating to witness the body heal naturally. The entire process is worth the time and effort.

I looked forward to Marc's herbs. I was curious to see what I could learn and what each day entailed. The information he shared with me seemed like a lot of daily work. I wasn't as prepared as I thought I was, however, not punching a clock was perfect. So, there's another reason the Universe led me to quit my punch clock. This healing crisis was already in the making, so what better way to heal than to be at home every day and nurture my body and, without any interruption. I knew a detox consisted of removing all things that no longer served you a purpose, and that included unhealthy emotions, "stinking thinking," physical waste and so much more. However, this process challenged every ounce of Goddess in me.

I thought healing from sexual abuse and depression was difficult, but this process was something different and astounding. I coached myself daily and thanked the Universe for my ability to do so. The average person wouldn't last a week under this program. It's highly challenging, very emotional and mental and just when you think you "got" it, the next week gets harder and harder. But, it's all worth it. I mentioned earlier that I received a scholarship for professional speaking school. Well, I must say, the Universe led my steps directly to Marc Haygood. It wasn't about the speaker's program as it was more about Marc's program. Marc's program saved my life and spiritually speaking, he is the reason I accepted the invite to the Entrepreneur Forum as well as the offer to attend NBC University. However, that does not discount James and Kara and all the other wonderful people I met.

CHAPTER EIGHT

Detox and Colon Cleanse

The 3rd week of June, and one week after I finished the turpentine and castor oil, I called Marc.

Phone rang
"Hello."
"Hey Marc."
"I'm ready to do your program now, but I won't have the money for another week or so."
"Oh, that's okay. I will still give you the products."
"Wow. That is awesome Marc. I appreciate you."
"It's cool. I trust you. So, when do you want to start?"
"As soon as possible."
"Okay, send me your email address."

For the next thirty days, I became more clear about what a detox and colon cleanse was. In the past, I juiced, fasted, did herbal detoxes exercised and most recently, turpentine. When my healing crisis began, I released fifteen pounds and felt better; however, something interfered with my body capabilities. In the past, I weighed one hundred and sixty-eight pounds, twice, might I add. The first time I was depressed after sexual abuse and blamed for it. The second time was during my pregnancy as I gained thirty-five pounds. Both of those times, I changed my diet, exercised and released all the excess waste plus a few more. What was different now? Why was I not able to heal my body via the same methods I used before? A part of treating the body is releasing waste, and over the past four years, I struggled with releasing and keeping the weight, waste off. Why? I will tell you why. When parasites eat your nutrition and release chemicals in your body, your body lacks what it needs to metabolize and excrete waste. Therefore instead of releasing waste, your body holds onto the waste as your elimination channels are incapable of discharging due to the toxic overload. What's more, your blood cells are incapable of carrying the proper amount of oxygen to your cells and organs.

My systems and especially my endocrine system, (hypothalamus, pituitary gland, thyroid, parathyroid, adrenal glands, pineal body, reproductive glands (ovaries and testes) and pancreas suffered in the past. I suffered from ovarian cyst and an ectopic pregnancy.

A cyst is filled with waste or toxic materials that are caused from the buildup of toxic waste in your body. I know doctors might say something else, but what is the purpose of testing the cyst after removing it. And in my case, it ruptured and put me on my ass. Painful was an understatement. All I remember was coming home from Chicago State University (CSU) and before I made it to the bathroom, I collapsed to the floor and awoke in the hospital. The doctor's diagnosed me with a ruptured ovarian cyst filled with pus-like fluid. Pus-like is directly related to white blood cells. My point, the cyst was filled with toxic fluid and based on my understanding, and during a woman's menstrual cycle, inside the fallopian tubes, an egg develops in a sac called the follicle. If the cyst doesn't open and release the egg, the fluid inside the follicle will form a cyst. Anytime fluid becomes hardened, or solid, it's waste and that is no different than a boil, or feces, as it is all toxic waste. What's more, the rupture can cause hemorrhage and severe pain due to sebaceous fluid spills and create chemical peritonitis (a potentially fatal inflammation of the abdomen's lining.) In essence, any form of fluid that leaks into the wrong place is considered waste or toxic. Isn't that what doctor's said years ago was the cause of cancer; when fluids leak over into an area of the body that it doesn't belong. That was all theory.

Everything we ingest becomes fluid and as mentioned when toxic materials compromise the protective barrier in the gut, that toxic fluid leaks over into the immune system eliciting a response that wreaks havoc on the body.

When parasites die off they release acetaldehyde and that chemical prevents red blood cells from transporting oxygen to your cells and organs. It doesn't take a rocket scientist to understand what happens when your cell or organ lack oxygen; try heart attack, stroke, pain, brain fog, and so much more. In the absence of oxygen, the function of organs is compromised, causing disease. What's more, the blood pH must maintain between 7.35 and 7.45. If there is even a tenth of change, the entire system or body becomes compromised making room for dis-ease and ultimately death.

My body was in slow death mode. I ran a 5k every other day and barely released one sweat. Sweat glands release toxins such as excess salts and other electrolytes including sodium, ammonia, cholesterol, and alcohol. The sweat glands are responsible for controlling the temperature, releasing pheromones as well as maintaining levels of salt in the body. When the body cannot sweat, it cannot cool itself, and that can lead to a heat stroke. What's more, according to Miller-Keane (1997), occlusion of the sweat ducts results in symptoms ranging from pruritus, scratch dermatitis and miliaria to very persistent inflammatory changes depending on the extent of the blockage.

Lastly, several things happen when you do not sweat. When you do not sweat, your body will not cool off; you fall victim to a host of opportunistic dis-eases, and you are at a higher risk of developing a skin infection or kidney stones. You may need more pain meds, wounds take longer to heal, and you may feel gloomy as sweating releases endorphins "feel good" hormone (Kulkarn, 2016). So, if I wasn't sweating, how serious is that? I was literally in the middle of a slow death. And it didn't start last year. I remember when I was about eight years old and had pin worms. My mother told me it came from overeating sugar. I learned later in life that the pinworms came from ingesting parasite larvae; eating gum or candy off the ground or meat products. What's more, I remember having ringworms several times. Ringworm is a symptom of yeast overgrowth. Sugar, fruit, carbs, meat, cheese, processed foods, sweet drinks, bread, boxed foods and so much more feeds yeast and worms. Candida albicans is a healthy flora of your mouth and intestines. Its job is to aid in digestion and nutrient absorption, but when overproduced, it breaks down the wall of the intestine and penetrates the bloodstream, releasing toxic byproducts into your body and causing leaky gut. Worms and an overgrowth of yeast cohabitated my body for the last thirty-eight years as I have experienced so much dis-ease. Today, after suffering all that I have in the past and current, I am convinced parasites and yeast is the reason dis-ease exists.

"Kelley, I sent week one. Did you receive it?"
"Yep, I got it."
"Make sure you read all of it."
"Okay, thanks, Marc."

Week one was very trying as the only foods I could eat was salads, a green apple a day, juices or other raw foods. I wasn't allowed to eat potato chips, nuts, eggs, meat, crackers or anything else that created an acidic environment. Week one also focused on detoxing my kidneys. I took at least twelve pills a day and several teaspoons or tablespoons of supplement powders. The bathroom became my best friend. When I wasn't running to the bathroom, I ran outside at the park. I recall doing my usual 5k at the park, and there was a forty foot hill that I ran up. As soon as I got to the top of that hill, I broke down and cried. I was angry at myself for treating my body so poorly for so long. The cigarettes, alcohol, meat, fried foods and everything I else I did to break my body down. As I cried and released those emotional toxins, something wonderful happened. Bobby Hutton song played in my ears. The lyrics said ... twenty years later, so here I am, searching for you.... I resonated with those particular words as it had been an exact twenty years since my first diagnosed with Psoriasis. Twenty years later, there I was on the top of a hill with my arms wide open and searching for healing. I smiled as I knew this was my time to release all emotions that no longer served me a purpose. I had to forgive myself for treating my body like crap. I cried, released, smiled and moved forward. I ran my 5k and noticed something else beautiful. I sweated as that was something I was not able to do. One week into the detox program, I released sweat and cried again; but tears of joy. That was a very poignant time as I knew right then and there; my body was on the road to recovery.

I ran daily in the summer and would not release any sweat at all. Even when the sun shined on me and it was hot, I did not sweat, so after one week of taking herbs, supplements, and flushing, something turned on in my body or started working again. I was pleased with the results. However, I was not happy with the cravings. I became present to the desires, and they were strong. It was like something told me to go and get a bag of potato chips or a slice of pizza or some chicken. I left the park and went directly to Family Dollar. I needed to pick up a few items, and on the way in, I texted Marc.

"Hey Marc, will it be okay to have a bag of chips?"
"If you want to feed the yeast, go ahead, they are going to have another party."
"I can't have one bag."
"You can, but I would encourage it."

I felt like an addict and bought a bag of chips anyway. I didn't understand why as soon as I ate them, the cravings went away. I felt guilty as I didn't realize how much damage one bag of potato chips was. The more starch I fed the yeast, the more they multiplied. I promised myself to make that bag, my last bag of chips. I also craved chicken, well not me, but the hijackers. In the middle of the night, I awoke to look for food like a zombie. So this is why I awoke in the middle of the night looking for food. I thought. It wasn't me. It was the yeast and parasites wanting food.

I didn't know how I would give up chicken. I gave up everything else, and all I wanted on occasion was a piece of chicken or a bag of chips. Now and then, I went into Mariano's and had some organic chicken breast. I thought the fact that it was organic, eating it was okay. Not at all. All meat products are acidic and ingesting anything acidic maintains an acidic gut, and that is precisely what parasites need. What's more, organic or not, according to the documentary What the Health, chicken has more fecal contamination on it than any other meat product. I may as well eat a piece of pork, just kidding. During the first week of the detox and cleanse, I had two party wings and one chicken breast. The other five days, I ate veggie dishes, salad, and green juices. I thought week one was hard. Week two was worse and required more mental toughness and physical strength.

By week two, I added the turpentine and castor oil back in my protocol to see if I would release any more worms. Week two focused on detoxing my liver, but I had to do a water enema first to ensure I got the entire bag in me. If I was not able to get the whole two quarts of water in my colon, then the coffee was a waste. So along with the herbs, I did a coffee enema for seven days. I hated the coffee enemas. Holding that coffee in was extremely mental, but after a few days of doing them, it became easier. In fact, the longest I kept it in me was about twenty minutes, and fifteen is the requirement. I was proud of myself. I had to take deep breathes continuously. I learned a trick before the seven days ended. That method was to tighten my stomach muscles, and for whatever reason, I was able to hold the coffee in longer. Some days after doing the water and coffee enemas, I felt drained, weak and sad. I wanted just to rest. After so many days and weeks, I was so sick of sticking that enema tip in my ass and tired of swallowing pills.

A part of my detox was to focus on the things I was grateful for as I was so distracted by what I didn't or couldn't have. I was angry and emotionally drained. I wanted to quit several times. I wasn't conditioned to eating only vegetables. I wanted bacon, (I didn't even eat bacon) macaroni and cheese, pizza, a sausage, egg McMuffin from McDonald's, steak, potato chips, ice cream, fried chicken, cheese and more cheese. I wanted everything I couldn't have and that left me feeling hopeless. What's more, I didn't want those foods, the yeast and worms did. Yes, they tasted good on my tongue, but that was as far as it went. I shifted immediately. I realized I needed to focus on what I had, not what I didn't have. I also had to keep in mind, the garbage I ate was the reason I was in a healing crisis. Each day I wrote down ten to twenty things I was grateful for, and that kept me in a mentally and emotionally great space.

I won't lie, I had a piece of chicken the second week, but only once for the entire week. I did better than the first week, and that was my goal, to just do better. I ate hummus and almonds from time to time and learned I couldn't eat those either. I was pissed off. But, I stayed focused on what I could have. Although it was only vegetables, I was grateful for that and water. I continued to run at least four days a week as I was excited to sweat. I also did foot detoxes.

"Hey Marc."
"Hey, hey. You look good. I can see a difference already."
Marc stopped by.
"You can? I feel different, well better. Something good is happening."
"Your skin. Your elimination channels are opening. Wow. This is amazing."
"I agree and guess what. I can sweat. I was not able to sweat before the detox. I cried when I felt sweat rolling down my head."
"Wow, you weren't sweating? Now that's amazing. I've heard some things but, never that. Wow. Your body was blocked. Wow. Well, it's over now."
"Yes it is, and I have you to thank."

Marc is such a humble and modest guy. He never takes credit for anything. Now although I did the work, his herbs assisted in healing my body. When I speak highly of him in his face, he never boasts or brags; he humbly says thank you. I knew there was a reason for our immediate connection and my connection to him.

Marc came by to render my foot detox, and the results were disgusting, but nothing short of amazing. After thirty minutes of soaking my feet, the water was at least five different colors, and they all meant something. In fact, my shoulder didn't hurt anymore after the detox and one of the colors in the water represented joint pain. I was completely amazed. I immediately released the emotion attached to the joint pain and shifted my thinking. Furthermore, I had other things to think about to be successful in healing my body and gratitude was one.

The second week was more tears, anger, stronger cravings and confusion. It was just too much "stuff" to take and not being sure of when to. Although I had all a complete schedule, adding the turpentine and castor oil back in the protocol became too much for me.

"Hello."

"Hey Marc."

"Hey, hey."

"I am baffled right now. The supplements seem like so much stuff to take, and I'm not sure when to add the turpentine and castor oil. I did it after the morning supplements and the coffee enema, but by the time I'm done, I'm starving and weak."

"Well, you can adjust the schedule as long as you get everything in you. It's okay to move some things around. "

"I can. Oh, thank goodness because this sh** is stressing me out. I feel so weak and tired."

"But remember this Kelley, this is what you go through during a detox. The body is trying to reset itself and, you're also not feeding the parasites so they are pissed off. But you have to stop eating the chicken. Parasites like flesh and blood. The yeast might like the sugar and starch but the parasites like the blood and flesh."

I cried.

"Marc this is so hard. Some days I want to give up, but I won't. I just feel so drained and confused. It's so much stuff to take and I feel like I'm not eating enough. I'm drinking more water than I ever have and there is never any room to eat. I want to eat." I cried.

Marc was silent on the phone as I expressed and released myself. He was a great listener.

"Well I know I can do it. I'm just trying to adjust mentally to this new way. I'm used to eating eggs and grits in the morning or a veggie omelet. This is so hard; having to give up foods so suddenly."

"Well, I'm glad you're able to release and share your emotions. That is really good."

"I'm sure you know by now that I am very transparent and sharing my emotions is very easy for me. I'm not holding this shit in. That's part of the reason I'm in this situation; harboring unhealthy emotions. So, you say the chicken feeds the parasites. That's really messed up. Giving up sweets isn't an issue I was never a fan of eating sugar. When I was eight years old, my mother told me I had pin worms because I ate too much sugar. So I stopped eating sweet foods. My problem is potato chips."

"How did you know you had pinworms?"

"My ass would itch badly and I stuck my pinky finger in and there were numerous worms on the tip of my finger. They were alive and moving."

"Wow. Are you serious?

"Yep, but I realized my mom wasn't telling the complete truth when I started school for medical technology. Worms or parasites come from ingesting the larvae (egg) in food. But you know that already. So, I have been a host for about thirty eight years. So imagine all the sickness I've endured. I recently learned that twenty million people in America alone are host for parasites and don't even know it. Some don't care to know it and some don't care to get rid of them. Well, this is my damn house and these little fuc**** have to get out. This is my body and I am taking control. So whatever I have to do to create optimal health that is what I'm going to do."

"I'm glad you mentioned optimal health. That's a good goal. Most people focus on the skin issue, diabetes or losing weight. Optimal health is great."

"Thanks Marc. It doesn't make sense to focus on healing my skin as if my entire body was healthy, like my organs, I wouldn't be in this situation. I just needed to vent. I feel better now. Every time I talk to you, I feel better."

"Thank you Kelley. I'm happy to assist you."

"Oh and real quick before we hang up. Just thinking back to when I first pulled those pinworms out and thereafter, I experienced a lot of dis-ease. I had allergies, sinus pressure, irritable bowel syndrome, inflammatory bowel disease, headaches, hemorrhoids, and gastroesophageal reflux disease (GERD). I also experienced diarrhea, constipation, bloating, heart burn, high cholesterol, high blood pressure, obesity, hypothyroidism, dry eyes, early stage heart disease and trigeminal neuralgia. Lastly, all the skin disorders that doctors have misdiagnosed me with, Psoriasis, Pityriasis Rosea and Lichen Planus. I am sure I am missing something, but I'm sure you get the point. Okay, well I guess I will go back to taking all this sh**." Marc and I laughed out loud.

"Okay Kelley, I will talk to you later. Bye."

I sucked it up and moved on. I released more emotional toxins and stinking thinking. I had power, but was no longer in control. My entire being was in a healing crisis as I had to tune in and start listening to what my body needed and not anything else. Whenever I craved, I merely talked to myself and moved through. I made it through week two without killing anyone and looked forward to week three. Week three was about detoxing the blood and lymphatic system. There were more and different supplements to take. However, by this time, I realized the detox worked so I stayed focus and created a plan that worked for me.

Most of the dis-ease I experienced were of unknown etiology or unknown cause. So, how does anyone define themselves as a doctor and have no idea where or how disease arises? There is a reason for the phrase "practicing medicine." Nowhere in the history of medicine or the history of medical education does it say "healing medicine." Why? The medical education system does not mention "healing" because allopathy medicine does not heal. Removing body parts, bleeding people and prescribing drugs does not constitute healing. Upon the diagnosis of Lichen Planus, Pityriasis Rosacea, Psoriasis, allergies, sinus pressure, inflammatory bowel disease, IBS, hemorrhoids, hypothyroidism, dry eyes, and trigeminal neuralgia, the doctor's told me the cause was unknown. So, if doctors have no idea where those dis-eases came from, why should we trust anything they say? We trust these random people with a doctoral degree because we've been programmed to believe the American education system is the "truth" as we've been brainwashed to believe that anything the European man teaches has to be the truth and the light. What's more, our deeply conditioned mindsets believe the healthcare system is about healing. Well, I digress. Some and if not all of these "doctors" are just as lost as the people who make appointments to see them. That statement is not to mistaken as an insult to doctors, but more so, a reality of what we live in today. For that reason, doctors have malpractice insurance. They do not know everything. Remember, I spent 23 years working alongside doctors as I am a member of the America Society of Clinical Pathologist. I do have a certain amount of respect for the healthcare industry as it employed me for many years and millions of other people, however, doctors should not play God with people's lives, and if they know the truth about parasites then it should be spoken.

I talked a doctor via telephone and asked if he would be interested in being a part of my documentary based on the journey you're reading now. His exact words were I have two doctor friends who almost lost their license for speaking out about candida and parasites. I love what you are doing, but I cannot help you. However, the information on my website is free to use. Lastly, if doctors are clueless about the etiology of disease, how would you know if worms and yeast aren't the reason for ALL disease? How would you know? Doctors obviously don't know, and after reading the first half of this book, you should now question everything your doctors tell you. Healing has never been in drugs and chemical as it has always been in nutrition, essentials oils, detoxifying the body and rodding out the septic tank or colon.

So far and during my detox, I released worms, yeast, old feces, unidentifiable objects, and now something called mucoid plaque. After much research, I discovered Dr. Richard Anderson and reached out to him via email. He coined the term mucoid plaque and is currently writing a book on health and wellness. After talking back and forth via email with Dr. Anderson, he permitted me to add a section on mucoid plaque from his book entitled Transformational Cleansing.   This segment is titled Mucoid Plaque.

The Creation of Mucoid Plaque
Mucoid plaque is a term that refers to the unnatural accumulation of intestinal mucins. Mucins are comprised of complex glycoproteins and have the ability to form gels and mucous and are key components in most gel-like secretions throughout the whole body.

I developed the term mucoid plaque, to describe this unnatural, but necessary emergency aid that has to happen in order to prevent severe damage to the intestinal wall caused by severe acids or toxins.

"Mucoid" is a general term for mucin, mucoprotein, or glycoprotein, which is the primary constituent of mucoid plaque.

"Plaque" designates a film or coating on a surface. In the stomach and intestines, mucoid plaque usually forms a continuous overlay that is composed of a structured fibrillary network and is arranged in layers, one layer upon another.

In the gastrointestinal tract mucins are secreted by gastric and intestinal goblet cells, which are present in the epithelium[1] wall of the stomach, small and large intestines. Mucin secreting goblet cells are also present in the respiratory system, sinuses,

---

[1] Epithelium is the thin tissue forming the outer layer of a body's surface and lining the alimentary canal and other hollow structures.

103

exocrine glands, sweat glands, upper respiratory tract, pancreatic ducts, nasal passages, lungs, liver/bile ducts, kidneys, outer layer of skin, mouth and vagina, lines epididymis, conjunctiva in the eyes, mammary glands and larynx. Numerous other organs have cells that secrete mucus. There main function of mucus is to protect the mucous membranes or the epithelium lining of these organs.

In a healthy environment, mucins serve as a microscopic lubricant for the intestinal lining. In an unhealthy environment, mucins are used as a protection against acids, toxins, and the toxins produced by pathogenic microbes, yeast, molds, fungus, parasites, heavy metals and pharmaceutical drugs.

While in the presence of these toxins copious amounts of sticky mucins are generated, layer upon layer. After the mucins have adhered to the gut wall, they coagulate and form a barrier that is intended to prevent acids, toxins pathogenic microbes from coming in contact with the epithelium wall. As mucins accumulate they compound with other elements such as food, fecal matter, acids, toxins, bacteria, parasites, heavy metals, pharmaceutical drugs, etc. These elements embedded in the mucoid plaque form an increasingly firm and toxic substance. Those who had followed the standard American diet and lifestyle, which, as you know, is acid producing and contains intense toxins, such as pesticides, chemical fertilizers, preservatives, toxic colorings, etc. and now worse than ever, GMO compounds, including glyphosate, which can alter the DNA of friendly bacteria. And may I remind you that once the DNA in your friendly have been altered, it is unlikely that you will ever be able to reestablish a normal healthy-producing microbiome and you will be subject to poor health for the rest of your life. Avoid GMO food at all cost. And, don't forget, if a food is not labeled organic you have a very high chance of it being GMO. Over 90% of corn, soy, wheat and canola oil are GMO. Even in some health food stores, particularly Whole Foods, the oils used in cooking and in their salad dressings are GMO.

It is common for mucoid plaque to form a continuous cover, arranged in layers, 2 and they can cover the glycocalyx3,4 of the small intestine. Coating the glycocalyx with mucoid plaque is not a good thing because just beneath the glycocalyx are our intestinal villi. This is where 90% of our food is absorbed.

When the villi is covered with mucoid plaque, then the digestive enzymes, including the pancreatic enzymes may not be able to make contact with the food you eat and your ability to fully digest and assimilate the nutrients you eat, become more and more limited.

It is important to understand that mucoid plaque develops only in an emergency for the protection of the gut wall. Without this protection the toxins could not only destroy the gut lining, but enter the blood stream; damage red and white blood cells and any tissues and organs that these toxins make contact with. To the best of my knowledge, this is the only reason that abnormal amounts of mucin accumulate into what we call mucoid plaque; gut protection.

Cystic Fibrosis is a dis-ease caused by excessive over secretion of tenacious, viscid mucins that accumulates and plugs ducts and glands of epithelial-lined organs.5 They call this excessive mucus mucoviscidosis, We could use the exact term

---

[2] J. R. Forstner, "Intestinal Mucins in Health and Disease," *Digestion*, 1978; 17(3), pg. 234-263.

[3] Glycocalyx: A thin layer of acid polysaccharides, particularly sialic acid, adherent to the outer surface of many cells. It may be the site of intense enzyme activity and also contains the surface antigens of the cell.

[4] The glycocalyx is designed to lubricate the structured fibrillary network of microvilli (the brush border), and allows for assimilation of nutrients. A continuous cover of mucoid plaque over the glycocalyx would obviously inhibit nutrient assimilation.

[5] Including the pancreatic ducts, the lungs, nasal passages, liver/bile ducts, kidneys, outer layer of skin, mouth, vagina, lines epididymis, conjunctiva in the eyes, mammary glands and larynx. When air passages become block, then it can be fatal.

for mucoid plaque, but conventional medicine prefers to just ignore the fact that the gastrointestinal tract in most people is full of mucoid plaque, which is tenacious, viscid mucus plugs, blocks and congests the epithelium wall.

Conventional medicine claims that cystic fibrosis is an inherited disease. I have a different opinion. What is likely to be inherited is the way they eat. The real causes, in my opinion are toxins or acids, which could be coming from fungus, yeasts, protozoa or chemicals from food or water. Any time our gut lining comes under attack, the mucins are secreted. These mucoid secretions form very sticky, gel-like, viscous mucus that forms a coating that can cover the entire gastrointestinal tract, which includes the stomach, small intestines and colon. This can also occur in any hollow organ such as the bladder and gallbladder and the others just mentioned.

In most cases, once the attack begins, it never stops as most people keep on doing the very thing they did that created the problem in the first place; mostly eating food and drinks that contain acids and toxins. The amounts of mucins that will be secreted will be determined by the degree of harshness, meaning the intensity of the acids or toxins and their amounts. This creates the abnormal accumulation of mucins that we call Mucoid Plaque.

Remember what I said about stem cells becoming a certain type of cell (bone, muscle, brain, etc.) that is determined entirely by the environment the cell is in? Stem cells will never become a bone cells if it is in a muscle environment. Similarly, different types of mucins are formed according to the chemical environment that surrounds the goblet cells, which will secret the mucins. So far, there 21 different types of mucins have been described. One of them is MUC1, which is commonly seen in the gut of people who have colon cancer. Other types of mucins may be formed in the presence inflammation. A different mucin may be formed in the environment dominated by colitis, and so on and so forth. The point is this: The type of chemicals in any area of our internal environment determines what is going to happen in every area of our body. As we continue to generate stress and eat toxic and acid-producing substances, layer upon layer of mucoid plaque builds barrier on top of a barrier, throughout the entire gastrointestinal tract, causing numerous issues depending upon how thick, how dense, and how toxic it has become.

Problems Caused By Mucoid Plaque
Constipation:
Conventional medical doctors state that normal is less than 3 BM's a week. Nothing could be further from the truth. I guarantee you that anyone who has that few of BM's has severely polluted their intestinal lining and destroyed his or her natural microbiome. This is to say; there health is slowly but surely, plummeting.

Mucoid plaque is probably the number one cause of constipation. Another cause is the incorrect microbiota (bacteria that are not friendly). We define constipation as having less than two or three bowel movement (BM) a day, depending upon how many meals a person has. Ideally, if we eat 2 meals a day, we should have 3 BMs a day; when we first get up in the morning and 20 to 30 minutes after a meal. Three meals a day is and we should have 4 BM's daily. This generally happens with truly healthy people and animals. This is Mother Nature's way. Many constipated people have reported that after the Cleanse, they have normal BM's exactly as I just described. Most people have to go through several Cleanses to achieve this ideal.

Constipation is a sure sign of trouble and an absolute sure sign that the body is accumulating more and more toxins, undigested proteins, fats, acids, etc. As long as a person has constipation they cannot become well and cannot achieve a high state of health, because their whole body is toxic and acidic. Our bowels are the number one most dynamic organ of elimination. When your bowel elimination slows down they become more and more filthy and this will stress your liver, kidneys, lungs and your largest organ of elimination, the skin. Blemishes, Psoriasis, acne and all your skin problems always begin in the bowels.

Dr. Jensen put it this way. When your bowels are dirty, your blood is dirty all the way into the cells. The very first day when I began studying with Dr. Jensen, he began to discuss one of his greatest secrets. He stressed the importance of keep the elimination organs clean. He taught that the kidneys, lungs, skin and bowels eliminate over 2 pounds of waste a day. He said that when any one of these four organs weakens that it would automatically force the other organs to work harder, which is to say, more and more toxic.

Soon after these organs become congested and less efficient, then all organs and cells will soon become congested and more and more toxic. Then waste products and mucus in the blood and lymph accumulate, and from this point these undesirable elements are forced into the cells. Constipation is also a sign that the natural to human microbiome has been significantly altered. You can be 100% assured of that.

The first thing every doctor should do for their patients is to assist them in eliminating constipation. No exceptions. No one can heal if they are constipated. The second most important act of every doctor should be getting their patients on a good health-producing diet. The third is to make sure they drink enough water. However, we do not see this happening because most doctors do not know how to treat constipation, nor do they know what a good healing diet is.

In my experience, the best way to eliminate constipation is to do a Cleanse such as I propose. I want to also say that the most important herb that can help strengthen in the intestinal wall is Cascara Sagrada, the scared herb of the Native Americans. However, one needs to combine Cascara with certain other herbs or it can be too harsh. No other laxative herbs can do this. Senna and aloe are purgatives, meaning way too strong, and over time they can weaken the peristaltic muscles that drive your bowel movements (peristalsis[6]).

Not being breast-fed usually causes constipation from the very beginning and this is caused by not having the correct microbiome. And, as you know just one round of anti-biotics will destroy the microbiome almost entirely. I cannot help wonder how many people who had normal BM's became constipated sometime after they completed their first round of antibiotics. Constipation can cause a stretching of the colonic wall, a ballooned wall, and this is a bad sign.

Other causes of constipation include:
- *Not drinking enough water*
- *Too much sodium chloride*
- *Pharmaceutical drugs*
- *Over use of laxatives*
- *Hypo and hyperthyroidism*
- *Depression*
- *Too much antacids*

Bowel Pockets, Diverticula, and Cancer Caused by Constipation

After our microbiome has been altered, then peristalsis becomes more and more inhibited, transit time of food through the alimentary canal becomes slower and slower, which causes greater and greater constipation. The more that peristalsis slows, food begins to rot before it exits and also loses its moisture, causing it to become dry, sticky, smelly, and sometimes hard. This rotting substance tends to attract pathogens and therefore inflammation, which can lead to IBS and other bowel disturbances such as colitis, Crohn's disease, polyps, colon cancer and many other gastrointestinal problems.

---

[6] The involuntary constriction and relaxation of the muscles of the intestine or another canal, creating wavelike movements that push the contents of the canal forward.

As constipation becomes more severe there will be greater and greater pressure placed upon the intestinal wall of both the small intestines and the colon. This pressure causes bulges and protrusions into the layers of mucoid plaque that form pockets. When these pockets, which are full of filth and highly toxic matter, are pressed beyond the gut wall, they are called diverticula. When diverticula become inflamed due to the incredibly toxic material being attacked by bacteria, then it is called diverticulitis. If these pockets of foul stagnant matter do not penetrate beyond the gut wall, then we call them bowel pockets, which by the way, are easily seen in the irises of the eyes.

At the beginning of the 21st century, diverticulitis was unheard of. As of 1987, bowel problems are so frequent that, according to the Merck Manual (the medical doctors' bible), diverticulitis is developing in 100 percent of the population and anyone who reaches age 90 will have developed diverticulitis.[7] Of course this is not true for those who refuse to follow the Standard American Diet (SAD), but it is true for about 90 percent of the Western world!

Diverticulitis is developing where we have the darkest and most filthy areas in our intestines. This is the perfect environment for worms and other parasites. It is in these places that yeast, bacterial infections and colon cancers develop. Cancer never ever develops without a cause.

Accumulating toxins, poisons, and free radicals gradually seep into the bloodstream and lymph system, settling in the weaker and more sluggish areas of the body; where unresolved emotional patterns reside. Consciousness is the precursor of all that happens. As these weak areas give way to the toxic

---

[7] Robert Berkow, MD, Editor-in-chief, "Diverticular Diseases" in *The Merck Manual of Diagnosis and Therapy, 15th Edition*, (Rahway, NJ: Merck, Sharp and Dohme Research Laboratories, Division of Merck and Company, 1987), 813-815.

overloads, disease develops into new dimensions. As Dr. Jensen always put it, "the name of a disease depends upon where the poisons settle."

Even when one succeeds in strengthening the weak area or somehow suppressing a symptom (as occurs when using drugs), the toxic flow from the bowel will back up into another area only to seek out a different place to break through. Dis-ease can only permanently be overcome when the cause is remedied (removed). The cause is always unresolved emotions. First there will be an emotional cause and second a physical cause. Sadly, "cause" is a word seldom used in conventional medicine. When we treat the cause, not just the symptom, we achieve success. Treating the symptom, which is what conventional medicine does about 98% of the time is always a temporary fix job.

I was discussing this with a fellow once who insisted there was no need to worry about cause. "When I get a flat tire I just fix it," he said. "I don't worry about the cause." I replied, "Would you try to fix the leak in the tire while the nail is still in it?" He said, "Oh, I see what you mean."

*Doctors do the very same thing when they cut out cancer in a colon or breast or blast the body with radiation, or poison the body with chemotherapy drugs. **They ignored the cause!** They do nothing to help the body heal itself. Patients go home and pray that it doesn't come back again, but what's stopping it from coming back? The original cause is still present! Seldom are they told to change their diets. Rarely are they given nutritional advice. Nor do many doctors even suggest to their patients the scientifically proven supplements that can relieve up to ninety percent or more of the side effects of chemotherapy. They just allow their patients to endure. So the patients go home and keep right on doing the exact same things they did that created their dis-ease in the first place. Does that make any sense? Is it any wonder that conventional medicine's cure rate for cancer is less than nineteen percent (which includes benign skin cancers) and*

up to eighty percent of that lucky nineteen percent will have their cancers return? [8] (Dr. Richardson Anderson. 2017)
   End Article

It was highly refreshing to not only read Dr. Anderson's section of his book, but also to connect with him as even as an M.D he understands that nutrition and the colon plays a key roles in creating and healing disease. Dr. Anderson also understands that most traditional doctors are not aligned with holistic doctors and for that reason and a few others; I needed his expert opinion on dis-ease and the colon. Dr. Anderson was more than willing to assist and share the information I requested.

I finally made it to my last week and was so very proud of myself. I released more worms, lots of yeast again, old feces and now mucoid plaque, but I was not convinced I was done with flushing and cleaning my sewage system. Your colon is no different than a sewage that holds waste until it backs up and wreaks havoc on your body/basement.

Everything we put in our mind, body, and soul will either break us or make us. With that said, if we all thought well, ate well, felt well and behaved well, doctors and the healthcare system would be obsolete. But, I highly doubt that will ever become the case. Mind brainwashing is just as real as a septic body.

Week four was for my digestive system, and I pooped more than I did the first three weeks. I also released more mucoid plaque, but this was worse than week three. I did my daily enema along with everything else and released. Everything that came out of me smelled like sewage. I grabbed my spoon, and there were three long worms at the bottom of the toilet. I wanted to puke it stank so badly.

---

[8] Numbers based upon data received by my office from the National Cancer Institute.

"Patrick. Oh my God, you have got to smell this. I smell like a damn sewage."

"Girl I don't want to smell that."

"Baby, please, just come to the bathroom door."

"Damn, damn, ugh, little ass sewage tank."

"I told you, and I just released three worms. This is just gross. I'm glad it's out of me."

The toilet water was black, and when I say it smelled of sewage, I meant every word. The entire fourth week, I released more mucoid plaque, worms, yeast, sewage smelling feces and some other stuff I could not identify. I was extremely disgusted and happy at the same time. I was detoxing my entire body. I felt phenomenal, happy, sad, grateful and mad all at the same time. My heart filled with joy as I came to realize that my body needed to heal and waited for me to say yes to health. Not only did I say yes to health and wellness, but I decided to share the progress of my journey.

I reached out to N'Digo Magapaper, "Eye on Chi," and sent the video of my skin. Torrence, the producer, was very interested in interviewing me. I greatly enjoyed sharing. I wore my white and black dress and noticed it was looser than last year when I wore it for my birthday. By this time and without even focusing on weight release, I had released about twenty-five pounds since I started my healing journey. The astonishing part was my stomach disappeared. I was excited to share my story as I was about the weight release; however, the journey was not an easy one and nor was it over.

I finished the twenty-eight-day detox, but according to the way my skin looked, I knew it would take more than a twenty-eight detox to heal my body. For me to obtain optimal health, I had to continue eating fruits and vegetables, detoxing, flushing, exercising and more. Opening my elimination channels was only the beginning of flushing out my entire being.

CHAPTER NINE

Worms, Worms, Worms

I decided to schedule an appointment with the University of Chicago hospital to have an ova and parasite (O & P) test done and to request some other testing. I wasn't interested in what the doctors had to say, or their opinions. On July 11, 2017, I took two worms in a glass jar to show it to the doctors. Pat and I patiently waited for the doctors to come into the room. A nurse came in and took my vitals and weight. My weight was down to 141lbs, blood pressure was 114/75, and my body mass index (BMI) was 23.63. My blood pressure was previously high, and around 150/99, my BMI was 31, and my weight was considered obese at 178 lbs. I was extremely confident in my body and what took place to make me sick.

Dr. Karl walked in, and I explained what I needed.
"How can I help you, Mrs. Turner."
"Well, several of the dermatologists here misdiagnosed me with skin disorders when in reality the issue was worms and yeast excreting toxins in my bloodstream. I have two of the worms that came out of me in this jar."

I arose from sitting on the patient bed, opened the jar and allowed Dr. Karl to look.
"Well, that's not something we can use. We have to do our own testing."
"I didn't expect you to use it. I expected you to look at it. I have several images of the worms that came out of me. Here are the images."

I selected camera on my S8 and opened the folder Optimal Health. I showed several images to Dr. Karl, and all he could say was, I'm not sure what that is, but we can do our own testing.
What the fu** is this dude talking about? It doesn't take a damn rocket scientist to identify a damn worm. These damn people are full of sh**. I thought.

"Let me take a look at your skin."

"My skin is fine. What you see is hyper-pigmentation and the after effect of the worms and yeast dying off and secreting over eighty toxins in my bloodstream."

"Are you sure you don't want to see a dermatologist."

"The dermatologist here misdiagnosed me so why would I want to see any of them. In fact, I am not interested in your suggestions. I just want to have an ova and parasite and a colonoscopy performed in case the O& P test misses the parasites. That test is only fifty percent accurate. I also have leaky gut so how will you test for that?"

"Okay, well let me talk to my boss, and I will be right back."

"This dude is unreal. I have a whole worm here, two of them and he ain't even interested in testing them or nothing. "

"Well, baby just get what you came here to get and don't even worry about him. You already know what's going on."

"You're right. I shouldn't have even come back in here."

Doctor Karl walked back in the room.

"I talked to my boss, and we can do the ova and parasite and the colonoscopy to check for the leaky gut. So, I'm going to write the order, and on your way out, someone at the front desk will schedule the colonoscopy and give you the instructions for the o & p. "

"Thank you."

Pat and I left U of C hospital and walked to the car. The next day I released and added some to the cup the receptionist gave me. I dropped the specimen off at U of C and went back home. As I waited for my test results, I sent Dr. Karl a message via *My Chart*.

---- Message ----
From: Kelley Porter-Turner
Sent: 7/31/2017 9:46 AM CDT
To: Dr. Karl
Subject: Question Regarding Test Results

Hi Dr. Karl

Do you all test for SIBO (Small Intestine Bacterial Overgrowth), if so, I'd like to have that test done as soon as possible. I'm not going to worry about the colonoscopy as I know I have parasites. I just released another worm yesterday, so I'm going to cancel that appointment. Please respond and let me know so I can schedule an appointment with you.

Response
Hi Ms. Porter, I see on 7/14 there was an OVA/parasite lab entered, please feel free to drop off a stool sample to the 3F lab at your earliest convenience. Please let us know if you need the supplies or just stop by any lab to collect a specimen cup.
Best-RN

---- Message -----
From: Kelley Porter-Turner
Sent: 7/31/2017 4:13 PM CDT
To: Nurse
  Subject: RE: Question Regarding Test Results

Hi,
It doesn't make sense to do another O & P as I've been holistically healing myself and have released numerous parasites and lots of Candida. I will just wait for the Colonoscopy to confirm the Leaky Gut. I would still like to know if U of C does the SIBO test.

Response
----- Message -----
From: Dr. Karl
Sent: 8/1/2017 3:16 PM CDT
To: Kelley Porter-Turner
Subject: (No subject)

Ms. Porter-Turner,
The O&P test was stained, and no organisms were seen. I agree with following up with the colonoscopy.
Dr. Karl

----- Message -----
From: Kelley Porter-Turner
Sent: 8/2/2017 11:32 AM CDT
To: Dr. Karl
Subject: RE:(No subject)

Dr. Karl
My question is does the University of Chicago do the SIBO test.
I'm not concerned with the misdiagnosis as I know what I have
released. Do I need to send more images? I want to know if you
all perform the SIBO test. Yes or No.

Ms Porter-Turner,
You do not need to send more images. I do not think testing for
SIBO is relevant at this point. I would continue with the current
plan of the colonoscopy, and we can touch base afterwards.
Karl, MD

I was done talking to Dr. Karl. Doctors can be so damn arrogant at times. What was so hard about him just answering my question about the SIBO test? What was the point of going around my request? I can only state the obvious, and that is doctors do not ever want you, the patient to be ahead of them in treatment. The idea of being wrong doesn't sit well with them. Being a doctor does not make you God and nor does it make you smarter than everyone. But it does make you more brainwashed.

It's one thing to brainwash humans, but it's a whole other thing when worms and yeast hijack your body. Up until the end of July, the longest worm I released was about eighteen inches long. I dug it out of the toilet stool and laid it on the sink. I went live on FB and exposed another creature living in my body. I wanted people to see what makes us sick and in fact, made me sick. If over eight billion people in the world have parasitic infections, why are doctors NOT treating the problem? Why are they focusing on the symptoms? Health care is a business, just like the food industry. It's not about nutrition, healing, and wellness. The bottom line has always been about capitalism.

The month of August was all about releasing worms, and it was unbelievable. Almost every day worms came out of me. I rarely saw any yeast. I was more knowledgeable about their behavior, like when they were irritated and restless and when they died. I was finally in control. I knew what the "itch" was and especially when there was no bug flying around or anything "on" my skin. That itch came from the inside as I felt the yeast and worms moving around under my skin. I also discovered that when my body temperature rose, and after that, I sweated, that was the death of them. I was excited to know that. So, I tested my theory. I took the turpentine while I worked at my home desk, and after that, I drank sixteen ounces of water. About forty-five minutes later, my body spiked. I sat still and waited patiently to see if I would spike again. About another thirty minutes, my body spiked again. About another hour from that, my body spiked again.

Okay, that's enough, flush them out of you. I thought. I grabbed my enema bag and added two quarts of distilled water. I inserted the enema tip into my rectum and allowed the water to flow into my gut. As soon as I sat on the toilet, three long worms came out of me. I was overly excited because I learned how to kill those suckers and knew when they died. Seeing the worms and yeast was proof that I never had an autoimmune disorder. Yes, my immune system was compromised, however, all of the symptoms I experienced were due to the yeast and parasites die off toxins released into my bloodstream. I was prepared to exterminate and eliminate all the aliens that hijacked my body. For the next two weeks, I ate vegetables, some fruit and herbs and especially ate cayenne, broccoli, cauliflower, garlic cloves, sunflower seeds, onions, coconut products and I took a 100 billion probiotic. The probiotic adds more good bacteria or "soldiers" to my gut. I was ready for war. For almost the entire month of August, I released worms and yeast every single day.

Our birthdays arrived, and this year, I promised to do something different and healthy, rather than the typical drinking, eating garbage and contributing to a slow death. I decided to do something fun, so Pat and I went to Go Ape and had a blast. My body didn't itch or burn. I felt good. We zip lined, walked several tightropes suspended in the air, swung from trees to rope walls and had to pull ourselves up, and we walked through several different obstacles all while being suspended in the air. We spent three hours completing obstacles, and the child and teenager in me were pretty happy. Shemar had a party with his female and guy friends. I preferred he went with me, but he didn't want to; teens.

Right around the second week of August, I made some essential oil suppositories. Patrick called me the research queen. I ordered books and read all I could about killing worms and yeast naturally as well as healing my gut. I created yeast and parasite suppositories by using several different essential oils and coconut oil as a base. To make the Candida suppository I used, bergamot, lavender, and lemongrass and eucalyptus globulus. According to Amelong (2017), bergamot breaks down mucus and toxic by-products produced by Candida and assist the body in repairing damaged tissue. Of the oils, bergamot is the most aggressive in treating intestinal infection and specifically Candida. Bergamot is also uplifting emotionally and is often used to relieve anxiety, stress, and tension. Lavender regenerates tissue while fighting off fungus (Amelong, 2017). Lavender improves mental functions, balances hormones and reduces inflammation. Lemongrass feeds healthy flora while restoring connective tissue and strengthening vascular walls. Lemongrass purifies the lymph system and reduces fluid retention. Eucalyptus globulus fights candida, and other related intestinal infections while promoting rapid healing, (Amelong, 2017).

The suppositories are like placing a bomb directly into your colon. The candida has no win. For the parasites, I used peppermint essential oil suppositories with coconut oil as a base. I also used tummy rub essential oil which is a blend of several oils. You can find the Tummy Rub on Amazon or Rocky Mountain Oils. The fun part about using the oils was whenever I felt the anal itch, I used the peppermint suppository, and the itch immediately went away. I did the parasite suppository for thirty days straight, alternating the peppermint and tummy rub blends. For

119

maintenance, I use the parasite suppository twice a week for a few months and the same with the candida suppository. I was amazed at how great the suppositories worked. Although this process may take a little longer than the traditional way of healing, I had the opportunity to watch my body heal itself, and that makes me proud. I respect and understand why my body is a temple. I didn't always treat it as such, but after this healing crisis, I love my body more than ever.

The number of worms that came out of me was incredible. When I say every day, I mean every single day. I released at least three to four different ones. I was amazed at how many I released as I was surprised at how the oil ruins a great pair of pants.

Shemar and I had dinner at the Cheesecake Factory in Orland. I had a vegan salad, and Shemar has a burrito. For whatever reason, I had to pass gas. Shemar should've been the one to pass gas considering he had beef and beans, but I did. I leaned over to my left side, and this gas must have lasted about four seconds. Now that may not seem like a long time, but for a fart, it is. When I got up, I felt something on my pants. I asked Shemar to take a look.

"Ma, there is a long streak on the back of your pants. It looks like you pee'd on yourself." Shemar's eyes widened.

"Are you kidding?" My eyes widened.

"No, I'm going to just walk behind you. I got you."

"Oh lord."

"Just walk Mama. I'm covering it."

"Shemar are you playing or are you serious?"

"Ma, I'm so serious, if you don't believe me just walk without me behind you."

"You play too much sometimes."

"I'm serious Ma."

We got up, and Shemar walked behind me. When we made it outside, I asked Shemar to video the area that he spoke of on my pants. When I looked at the video, I was so grateful my t-shirt was too long. I untied it in the front and hid my behind as we walked through the mall and to the front where my car was parked. I had no idea the oil was going to come back out, I mean, at least not that much. From that day on, I prepared myself for visits to the bathroom as if I had to release. Speaking of the bathroom, later that evening and after my flush, I released a worm that had to have been about 2 feet long or more. I grabbed my toilet spoon, and as I pulled the worm towards the top of the toilet, I didn't see an end to it.

"Patrick! Come quick! This mofo is long as hell. I don't see the end to it. What the hell? This little nigga has to be about two feet long."

Pat came running in the bathroom and was just as amazed as I was.

"Wow! What the hell. That's a damn alien. I'm going to call your ass the alien lady."

I laughed.

"Let me see if I can get it out of the toilet without breaking it. It's too damn long. Damn it. I didn't want to break it. Well, I will just lay it on top of some tissue on the sink."

It was way too long to pull it out the toilet without breaking it. I was utterly grossed out, and that thing looked like an alien for real. It looked like a pile of worms, but, was one worm. Of course, I stared at it for several minutes as I wondered where his big ass hid all this time. I was happy to release it. In fact, I didn't release any more worms for another two weeks or so. My body worked, and I was excited. All the hijackers I released was proof of what made my body sick. Not only did I exterminate and eliminate numerous worms and yeast, when I started back in June, I took almost thirteen supplements a day, daily enemas and so much more. At this point, I only took four supplements and used the suppository. When the body is in position to heal, it will do so. You cannot load the body up with white sugar, white, flour, white bread, white pasta, processed foods, meat, GMO's, fried foods, cheese and other toxins and expect the body to eliminate regularly. Your gut will become blocked, dis-eased and you will become sick. Once your stomach is waste-filled, you cannot expect your organs to receive the nourishment they need to function. It's a domino effect. A toxic colon means a dis-eased body. That was my case. Waste like worms, yeast, mucoid plaque and so much more filled my bowel. How was my body going to exterminate and eliminate anything when it was a septic tank that compromised my immune system and organs?

The moment my elimination channels were detoxified and open, every opening on my body became a way out. During the middle of the night, I felt some discomfort in my chest area and not like your typical chest pain. The pain was like heartburn, but without the burn. I also felt nauseated, I took some deep breaths and went back to sleep. Later, when I awoke, the discomfort was still there. It felt like something was stuck in my upper chest area or closer to my throat. I gagged as I wanted to puke. I went to the bathroom, and the force was strong, but nothing came out. Over the next 72 hours, the discomfort in my chest just lingered. I felt nauseous.

At the suggestion of Marc, I decided to take some licorice and marshmallow root. I opened the capsules and poured the powder directly into boiling water and drank eight ounces daily. After day three, I felt that powerful feeling again in my throat. My body wanted whatever it was out of me. I coughed and gagged. My eyes filled with water as I felt sick. After about ten minutes of gagging, I threw up yeast directly out of my mouth. I was grossed out. I thought that was it and more came. Thick white and tan stringy stuff filled the toilet. I let it sit there before flushing to see if it would behave like yeast. When yeast is in water, it tends to grow leg-like structures. I waited about fifteen minutes, and the leg-like structures were there. I took a picture and videoed it. That was grosser that eliminating from my anus. I brushed my teeth and mouth for about five minutes.

The one thing I noticed since puking the yeast was that crackle noise within my lungs was gone. Whenever I laid down at night or anytime, I heard a single crackle or gurgle like noise in my chest area when I inhaled. I am happy to know I eliminated that waste. I also noticed my body no longer burned.

I also noticed when my body needed to eliminate or after the die-off, I only perspired around my forehead. In comparison to what the die-off symptoms were before, that told me that the yeast and parasites were close to total extermination. I wasn't in the complete clear, but I worked my ass off to get to this point, and there was no turning back.

My body is now capable of exterminating and eliminating all things that no longer serves it a purpose. Once you release the emotional and mental toxins, the physical body aligns itself. As mentioned in Chapter one, some of the emotions I dealt with before this healing crisis was worthlessness, anger, and sorrow. Once I acknowledged those feelings, I was able to look at the source, nurture myself and start the process of healing. In essence, I had to eliminate those emotional toxins, and I did so by crying and forgiving myself. I had to excuse myself for mistreating my body for so long when I knew better. I knew the damage smoke, meat, alcohols and processed foods caused. But, since I was conditioned as a child, eliminating these things from my life took time. Worthlessness, anger, and sorrow are three very familiar emotions to my DNA. Everything we ingest, think and feel becomes liquefied. Feelings are no different than food as everything is energy.

CHAPTER TEN

Healing Crisis Symptoms

I didn't realize when my body burned, itched, and broke out that it was my body fighting back. I thought something was attacking my body. In fact, I thought something tried to come through my skin, and that may have very well been a part of the issue. However, my body reacted to something. My body fought to remove the worms and yeast, and they fought back. My body wanted to heal, and unfortunately, my skin took the most significant hit. Die off symptoms are merely the body's reaction to chemicals released in the body and the bodies way of trying to remove these unhealthy and foreign chemicals.

Some of the "die off" symptoms I experienced over the past year were hives, allergies, congestion, sinus pressure, flu-like symptoms, itching, and headache, fatigue, burning; like hot flashes, sweating, insomnia, brain fog and joint pain. Some of the dis-ease or symptoms I experienced due to the chemicals released into my bloodstream were hypothyroidism or imbalanced hormones, emotional instabilities, Psoriasis, Pityriasis Rosacea, Lichen Planus, hemorrhoids, and dry eyes. The commonality between all of those symptoms or dis-ease is that they stem from worms and yeast toxins released into the bloodstream. But keep in mind, my body's response is what ultimately creates the healing crisis as in the absence of toxins; the body has no reason to react. Billions of people all across the world suffer from the same issues and have become conditioned to that lifestyle. The "symptoms" have been there so long that people claim disease as "theirs" and do not question anything. I can't judge as that was me. I used phrases like my sinuses, my allergies, just as people do today. Since I was about eight years young, I remember hives popping up in my face during the off-allergy season like in the winter time. I also recall sinus pressure and congestion that doctors categorize as disease and we all fell for it.

According to Miller-Keane (1997), a symptom is any indication of disease perceived by the patient. A disease is a definite pathological process having a characteristic set of signs and symptoms. It may affect the whole body or any of its parts, and its etiology, pathology, and prognosis may be known or unknown (Miller-Keane, 1997). So, a disease is a state in which the body is no longer in a healthy state. With that said, is it safe to say that worms and an overgrowth of yeast are dis-eases and an unnatural state of being for the body? I believe so seeing as though humans are not born with worms excess yeast and intestinal worms. So, what are the symptoms of yeast overgrowth and worm infestation? The same ones that doctor diagnose as dis-ease are the same symptoms that classify as die-off signs.

As a Personal Development and Transformation Coach, I deal with root issues as scratching the surface has never helped anyone. The symptoms are considered the surface and the worms and yeast are the root. If doctors continue to treat symptoms, dis-ease or healing crises will never cease.

Some other symptoms of yeast overgrowth and the parasitic infestation is anal itching, ear itch, creepy crawly under the skin, and grinding your teeth. I experienced all of those and most of us do and believe they are just some ordinary phenomena like ear wax in the ear, an invisible bug, stress, and a dirty ass. I digress as the healthy body does not present symptoms of any kind, NONE. However, somewhere along our journey, we have been conditioned to believe that sickness is normal, and as long as they don't cause us significant issues, we accept them as ours, continue taking medicine while the body slows down and eventually dies.

I mentioned the itch earlier, and how we scratch and slap our skin assuming something crawled on it. However, have you ever wondered if that itch came from the inside? Or are we so unaware of the truth that we believe a fly landed on our skin in the heart of the winter? Not only did I experience that deeply rooted itch at the beginning of my crisis, but I feel them little creatures crawling and dying underneath my skin as I write, at this very moment. However, the way my body is set up, I am healed. Although this chapter deals with die-off symptoms, I wanted to share this article I found on Google as it relates to your gut and healing, and written by Kat Maede.

Gut Microbiome. Kat Meade

What's the first thing you consider as the cause of your fatigue or those mid-afternoon energy slumps? What comes to mind when you're constipated, forever catching other people's colds, or when you're battling hourly mood swings? Do you know what's underneath your constant sugar cravings?

I'll bet it's not your gut that comes to mind…right?

Don't feel bad! That was me some years ago too! I had no idea! It wasn't until I did my deep dive into holistic health that I was able to get firsthand the impact my diet, along with some other lifestyle stuff (stress, medications, etc.) had on my gut. Consuming, dairy products, grains (most, of course, with gluten), incorrectly combining certain foods, along with eating sugar and processed foods left me tired, sluggish, and sometimes downright irritable. It took just one cleanse based on an elimination diet for me to connect so many dots and see the profound effect that food and lifestyle choices can have on digestive health and gut function, both of which are integral to overall wellness.

Your gut is so much more than just your stomach digesting food. In fact, many people are shocked to learn that their microbiome – the intestinal gut ecosystem – is critical to their overall health. Put simply; your gut is your gateway to vibrant, thriving health. When digestion is impaired, it impacts all the systems in the body, not just the digestive system. You might call your gut your Grand Central Station. Quite honestly, you can eat as clean as possible, exercise daily, keep stress under control, and get enough sleep, but if your gut is out of balance, you're not going to feel or be on top of your game.

Thankfully, many researchers are beginning to see the clear connection between the gut and one's health. They are finally recognizing the importance and need to restore the integrity of the gut's ecosystem. This is an incredible and exciting move forward for 21st century medicine, **especially because so many diseases that are seemingly unrelated to the gut – such as Eczema , Psoriasis, acne, skin disruption, impaired thyroid, obesity/diabetes, mental illness, autoimmune diseases, and cancer – are often initiated by gut dysfunction and inflammation.**

"All disease begins in the gut" – Hippocrates

Gut Health – Breaking It Down
Having a healthy gut is truly the foundation to your wellness, inside and out. Your digestive system is made up of the hollow organs of the gastrointestinal (GI) tract, which includes the mouth, esophagus, stomach, small and large intestine. It also includes the solid tissue organs: the liver, pancreas, and gallbladder.

The organs of the digestive system, together with your gut flora, work with a web of nerves, hormones, bacteria, and blood to keep you healthy and balanced.

Let's take a closer look gut health:
Microbiome
- *Bacteria in the GI tract are also called your gut flora. Collectively, the ecological community of symbiotic and pathogenic micro-organisms that share the space of our body, whether in health or illness, are call the microbiome.*
- *The microbiome helps us digest food.*
- *They also regulate hormones, help eliminate toxins, and produce vitamins, plus other healing compounds that keep your gut and your body healthy.*
- *This ecosystem of friendly bacteria must be in balance to do their crucial work.*

Gut-immune system

127

- *Eighty percent (yep, 80%) of your immune system resides in your gut.*
- *Your immune system and the rest of your body are protected by a lining that functions as a barrier to the toxic environment in your gut*
- *If that barrier is damaged, you may experience nutritional malabsorption or have a compromised or overactive immune system that triggers inflammation, which can become chronic and systemic.*

- *Gut protection is key to defending your body from being invaded by unfriendly critters, such as parasites, bad bacteria, viruses, etc.*

Gut-Brain axis – your gut's nervous system

- *The gut system actually contains more neurotransmitters than your brain and is often referred to as the "second brain."*
- *Messages constantly travel back and forth between your gut-brain and your brain; when those messages are interfered with in any way, **your health will suffer.***
- *The majority – 70-80% – of your happy, feel-good hormone, serotonin, is produced in the gut. If your gut is out of balance, you'll feel out of balance; without the feel-good hormone, mood disorders, such as depression and anxiety, can manifest.*

My gut has been unhealthy more than ¾ of my life

Detoxification

- *Your digestive system is designed to remove toxins and acid wastes that are by products of metabolism.*
- *If things get backed up –constipation – your body will become toxic and your overall health will suffer.*

Digestion

- *The digestive and gut system is designed to break down all the food you consume into simple usable parts and then delivers the vitamins and minerals, as well as fats, amino acids, and glucose to the bloodstream to nourish your body and brain.*

- *If your digestive system in not functioning or is out of balance and your body isn't absorbing nutrients, you can become nutrient deficient even though you are eating the right foods.*

Our modern lifestyles are the perfect breeding ground for the harmful bacteria that kill off the good guys. Every day, we traumatize our guts with poor food choices, medication, stress, etc. The overgrowth of the harmful bacteria also impedes your immune system, promotes illness, infection, and imbalances that weaken and further inflames your entire organ system.

Common symptoms of toxic/gut imbalance
- *Low energy*
- *Sluggish metabolism*
- *Weight gain/inability to lose weight*
- *Cravings*
- *Poor sleep quality*
- *Skin issues*
- *Mood swings, depression, anxiety*
- *Brain fog and memory problems*
- *Low libido*
- *Low immunity; chronic colds and flu and other infections*
- *Food allergies, intolerances and sensitivities, Celiac disease*
- *Digestive issues, including gas, bloating, constipation, IBS, GERD, colitis (including ulcerative colitis)*

Thriving health begins in the gut (Kat Maede, 2016.}
End Article

Do you notice the similarities in the symptoms of a toxic gut and what I experienced? I have experienced everything listed in the common symptom area and more. What's more, many of those symptoms mimic die off symptoms. Either way, when the gut is toxic, so are the cells, organs, systems, and body. The one sign that drove me nuts was insomnia.

I distinctly remember awakening in the middle of the night as I never understood why. Not only did I awake in the middle of the night, but I also went directly to the refrigerator seeking something. The significant part about it was, whatever those parasites and yeast wanted, it wasn't in my fridge. However, before my transformation, I awoke in the middle of the night and ate chips or a hot dog. Why? Why was I awake like a damn zombie in the middle of the night seeking and eating? Why was I not able to sleep?

After reading Aston's article on parasites, I wanted to share it with you as well. I mean it is one thing to have symptoms, but to have eliminated hundreds of worms from my body along with enormous amounts of yeast, the information I researched and read was imperative to my journey of healing. I think you will find this next article just as fantastic as the other articles. What's more, every symptom discussed I experienced, and now I understand the burning sensation that I felt.

10 Key Signs of Knowing Whether a Parasite is Present in the Body Include: David Aston

Let us discuss in general the path of a parasite infection in the body before moving on to the distinct symptoms. When the parasite infection is acute, abdominal distress in varying degrees may be experienced by an individual. This distress includes diarrhea, fluid loss and burning sensations.

Visible evidence of an infection is seldom present at this stage of the problem. It is possible to go a step further and state that the parasites do not always appear in the specimens tested in laboratories. Guess they are pretty good at hiding themselves!

A parasitic infection will move from the acute to chronic stage. At this point apart from the diarrhea; constipation, intense burning, bloating of the abdomen, cramping and sudden urges to eliminate, become part of the symptoms. There can be sudden food cravings, weight loss, irritable bowel syndrome, blood sugar fluctuations and mal-absorption of nutrients from foods consumed. The problem when untreated can continue to manifest

130

itself through acute itching of the body; sleep disorders, skin sensitivity, anxiety and depression.

*1. **Immune Disorders**: Parasites are like leeches, sucking the nutrients out of the body. This results in an immune system that is forced to operate on a lower supply of essential vitamins, minerals, nutrients and energy sources. The parasite is capable of stimulating the production of the body's defense mechanism immunoglobulin A. Overstimulation results in exhausting the supply leaving the body wide open to various bacterial, fungal, viral and other attacks.*

*2. **Sleep Disorders:** Parasites, especially the ones that prefer to nest in the intestinal tract, can cause a host of sleep disorders such as insomnia. Parasites affect the nervous system as well, giving rise to sleep disorders. All through the night, the body is hard at work eliminating toxins through the liver. Parasites are known to upset this routine, changing the body's rhythm. Some parasites cause a great deal of itching around the anal area, disrupting sleep and causing discomfort to the person.*

*3. **Bruxism:** Bruxism is the medical term given to teeth grinding; clenching teeth tightly together or grinding the back teeth over each other. At first glance, the connection between teeth grinding and parasites may not be clear. Teeth grinding, clenching and gnashing of teeth happens at night when the person is asleep. This happens due to anxiety and restlessness caused by the parasites releasing waste and toxins into the body.*

The weird part about the teeth grinding is that I had no idea I did until I went to the dentist over ten years ago. My dentist told me based on the looks of my teeth; I needed a guard because I grind my teeth at night. Apparently, there was something about my teeth that indicated that. At any rate, I paid a few hundred dollars for mouth guard and still have it. The dentist never said why I grind my teeth or gave me any indication that she knew why. Now I know why.

4. Skin Problems: *Parasites that attack the intestinal tract cause inflammation and considerable skin irritation due to the release of hormones into the body. These in turn irritate the skin causing rashes, hives, Eczema and other forms of allergies to attack the skin. Another problem with an inflamed intestinal tract is that digestion of certain foods becomes difficult. Undigested foods produce increased eosinophils levels that inflame the tissues causing allergic reactions. Some parasites cause sores, swellings, lesions and ulcers to break out.*

5. Irritable Bowel Syndrome: *Irritable bowel syndrome or IBS is one of the more common signs of a parasitic presence in the body. Intestinal parasites dig in and fix themselves to the walls of the intestines. This leads to inflammation and irritation of this area that soon leads to cramping and spasms and intestinal blocks. Mal-absorption of nutrients from food follows, and some foods become hard to digest.*

I experienced IBS when I was about 30 as I remember it during the tie I worked for Rush North Shore hospital in Skokie, Illinois. Painful was an understatement as I was incapable of walking and was taken down to ER in a wheelchair. Unfortunately, I never got a solid diagnosis and continued to suffer as the years passed.

6. Stomach Disorders: *Parasites attack the human body in various ways including causing constipation. Worms are parasites and can actually block the passage of nutrients into the body, and waste from exiting the body at various points in the digestive system. Parasites can attack the bile duct and intestines causing the digestive system to malfunction. When this happens, the normal bowel movements are hampered causing constipation. Another stomach problem caused by parasites is flatulence. Parasites enjoying residence in the upper small intestinal region cause inflammation of the area. This leads to a bloated feeling that is very discomforting; add to that the formation of gas. All of which is compounded by the consumption of certain foods that are hard to digest.*

7. Diarrhea: *Parasites generally attack the lining of the intestines, but also have the potential to attack all other parts of the body. All through a parasitic infection, a variety of abdominal problems prevail in distressing regularity. Watery, loose stools that are painful to eliminate is one of the more common abdomen problems. The fluid loss if unattended, leads to severe dehydration. To top it all, several parasites produce a chemical called prostaglandin that leads to the loss of chloride and sodium from the body, causing in turn diarrhea.*

8. Body Ache: *As parasites are migratory rather than stationary, they sometimes tend to become enclosed in a cyst like manner in the muscles and even joint fluids. The result is irritation which is the lesser end of the problem; pains and an aching follows that is often mistaken for arthritis. Pain in the muscles and joints may also be caused by the immune system's response to the parasites invading the body.*

I have experienced joint and muscle pain that doctors were unable to determine the cause. I was also prescribes muscle relaxants for my unexplained muscle pain. Unfortunately the pain returned over the years.

9. Chronic Fatigue: *There is no doubt that parasites deplete the body of vital nutrients leading to exhaustion at mental, physical and emotional levels. When parasites invade the body causing the mal-absorption of vitamins, minerals, fats and carbohydrates, the body is left drained of energy. This inevitably leads to acute exhaustion, depression, concentration difficulties and general apathy.*

Back in 2014, when I was diagnosed with hypothyroidism, I slept at least 16 hours a day and had absolutely no energy. The doctors blamed my thyroid as the test results were subclinical-meaning not within diagnostic range- and they prescribed a pill. I took levothyroxine for three years and today I am no longer on any medicine as my thyroid is normal.

10. Other Symptoms: Parasites can cause a number of other problems apart from the ones previously listed by which an infection may be determined. Some of these include: food sensitivities; anemia – iron deficiency; excessive number of bacterial or viral infections; excessive weight gain or loss; restless anxiety; itching of the ears, nose and anus; forgetfulness; slow thought process; excessive eating but continue feeling hungry or alternatively loss of appetite; lethargy; drooling during sleep; problems with menstrual cycles for women and sexual dysfunction for men; numb hands. These are all possible symptoms of the problem (David Aston, 2015)
   End Article

In essence, all nine of the symptoms listed in Aston's article were mine at one point. Although I am healing my skin naturally, I haven't had any more breakouts. I have also experienced several of the symptoms mentioned number ten.

I shared these articles as I want you to understand that there is so much information in the world, that there is no way you should suffer physically, mentally or emotionally. Even if you are not one of those people who like to research, you have people like me who are willing to share my experience to help you. What's more, even if you refuse to pick up a book and read, YouTube University has tons of videos that you can watch on healing, and if that doesn't work; you have Coach Kelley as my work is my purpose.

Every symptom I experienced was really at the emotional or spiritual level. Sure, all the signs discussed in the book were physical, but metaphysically speaking, my unhealthy and toxic emotions played a significant part in the physical manifestation of dis-ease. Hives represent small hidden fears. I've experienced hives since I was a child and yes there was always fear present. My household was very abusive and violent and so I was sometimes afraid to go to sleep at night. Allergies represent denying your power. I always said I was allergic to people, but in the scheme of things, I dismissed my power. Constipation represents holding onto old ideas and stuck in the past. Well, I've already expressed to you how I was stuck in my childhood when I met my husband, and in a more current past regarding my husband's behaviors. Sinus pressure represents irritation to someone close. I haven't experienced any sinus pressure in over six years, but when I did, I dated my son's father. I was irritated by his deceptive behaviors and sarcastic mouth.

The flu represents responding to mass negativity and beliefs or believing in statistics. I had the flu when I was about twenty-one years young, and during that time, I dated a married man as I also thought I was a homewrecker for doing so. Today, I understand a happy home won't permit outsiders to invade their space. Itching represents desires that go against the grain or unsatisfied and remorse; itching to get away. During my healing crisis, I wanted away from Shemar and Patrick and not because they did something, but, I wanted to be free of taking care of everybody else and focus on me. I was very unsatisfied and filled with remorse. Before this particular day, I felt remorseful as I wanted a divorce the year prior and regretted that I didn't move forward. Today, I am happy I stayed with my husband. A headache represents self-criticism. I've had one in the last ten years, and that one was when I went to ER for my skin. I criticized myself a lot as didn't approve of my skin. I'm over that. My skin is beautiful and so am I. Fatigue represents boredom and resistance. I can admit during my fatigue days, I was bored as hell and did not like working as Medical Technician anymore. I resisted the idea of happiness with a job I hated. The burning represents anger or burning up. I can go back to hating and feeling angered about staying with Pat when his experience with alcohol was indifferent and unhealthy. That's over now. I am not sure about the excess sweating, but emotionally speaking, I can assume it means to release those things that no longer serve you a purpose. Insomnia represents fear and not trusting the process of life. Well, I'm happy to say I sleep very well at night. There is no reason to elaborate on all of the symptoms I experienced as I believe I made my point. In essence, all that negative energy weighted heavily on my body and manifested itself according to my emotions. When the spirit speaks loud, and we choose not to listen, the physical body suffers.

I dealt with die-off symptoms or a toxic gut for over thirty-eight years. At around eight years old, I experienced chicken pox and hives. By the time I was a teenager, I had experienced inflammatory bowel disease, diarrhea, bloating, constipation, weight gain, and cravings. By my early twenties, I experienced skin issues, mood swings, depression, and anxiety. By late twenties and early thirties, I experienced low energy, more cravings, brain fog and memory problems, as well as irritable bowel syndrome. By my late thirties, early forties, I experienced, low libido, sluggish metabolism, weight gain and inability to lose weight, poor sleep quality. Lastly, over the past five years, I have experienced food allergies, intolerances and sensitivities. So, it is safe to say that my gut and body has been toxic for a very long time. So, when you look at my skin, you're looking at years of emotional and physical toxins. And believe it or not, I am grateful I have this opportunity to share it with you. I only speak health and wellness into my life, but I could very well suffer from cancer right now. Please understand I am very grateful to Mr. Parasite and Ms. Yeast. Their presence has brought nothing but light to my life. Now, I pay close attention to my body, what I eat and any symptoms that might arise. Recently, I tested my gut with a few foods. Pat and I went out to have a salad, and I added five pieces of thin, square cheese. Two days later, I had a horrible case of gas. That amount of gas triggered a time in my life when I worked my first job in the Healthcare Industry. I was about twenty-one and worked for Dr. Cyrus Akrami over on 91st and commercial. I was a medical assistant. An older black man with a gray beard needed services from Dr. Akrami. He was about six feet tall with a big belly, short grey and black afro and matching beard and mustache.

"Good Morning, how can I help you today Mr. Washington."
"I cannot stop passing gas."
"How long has this been going…

136

"Excuse me."

"How long...

"Excuse me.

"Okay, how many days?"

"Excuse me. I can't stop farting. Excuse me. I've been farting ... Excuse me ... for about two days now."

I sat very close to Mr. Washington, and he farted about fifty times in about five minutes.

"Excuse me. Oh God. Excuse me. This is driving me nuts. How can I stop it?"

"Mr. Washington the doctor will talk to you about that. I need to take your blood pressure, temp, and pulse."

"I'm so sorry."

"It's okay."

On the inside, I laughed so hard I almost burst out in his face. While he farted, I laughed. I thought it was hilarious.

"Your blood pressure is high, but everything else is normal."

"I know. I didn't take my medicine this morning. I'm so stressed out from farting. I don't even want to go around anyone, as they stink badly."

Yes, the hell they do. I thought.

I opened the door to air the room out. I was about to suffocate in that room. Those farts were deadly and loud.

"Do you have any pain with them?"

"No, no pain; just driving me nuts."

"Okay, well, Dr. Akrami has two patients ahead of you."

"Okay. Excuse me. Excuse me."

I walked out the room and went directly into the bathroom. I had to contain my loud laugh. I cried in that bathroom. My stomach felt like it wanted to burst. I pulled myself together and moved on to the next patient.

That was me after eating that cheese. The five cubes probably amounted to a quarter of a slice of cheese. My goodness, for almost two days, I ripped the runway. That's what Pat called it. They were loud, long and stunk like hell. The light finally clicked in my head. Farting is a symptom of a toxic colon, and the smell is as well. I immediately flushed my colon with a lemon enema for three days straight and used my colon sweep supplement. In healthcare, professors taught a fart is nothing but undigested food. I guarantee I will never eat cheese again. I'd instead stand in a corner and hold an encyclopedia for an hour than create that type of misery.

A week later, I tested my body with fried catfish. You're probably wondering why. Well, experiences are always the best teacher. It is one thing to listen to folks tell you what you should or should not eat, but it's another to eat something and suffer the consequences.

How many times have you ate something and your stomach spoke to you. You developed gas, bloating, constipation, headache or some other "symptom" that you assumed simply came from eating. Well, eating some "thing" definitely triggered your body's reaction, but why. The foods we ingest are man-made and not from the source. The source is the Universe, God, the Infinite or whatever you choose to call the source. The foods we eat are not from the earth as they are from the laboratory or factory. That will explain your symptoms, healing crisis, or disease. We are ingesting chemicals all day every day. Practically everything white is bleached. Can you imagine what bleach does to the digestive and immune system? Can you imagine what Round-Up does to the digestive and immune system? Remember, if our gut "feeds" our cells and organs, imagine what our cells and organs are absorbing; chemicals, so why do you think I you have symptoms? Nothing is hereditary as every disease stems from toxicity. Whether it is toxic emotions or colon, you created it, so you can now un-create it, just as I did.

I tried some fried catfish, and my gut felt horrible. The gas was just as bad as when I ate that cheese. Catfish used to be my favorite fish until my introduction to salmon. After eating that one piece of fried catfish, I acknowledged several things. The fish was probably deep fried in canola oil, dumped in white flour, and died a miserable death. What does that mean? I ingested unhealthy fats, emotions, and bleach. All the symptoms I experienced were my body reaching out for help. Symptoms are not normal. I know you think they are since you have lived with them for so long. But, I hate to be the one to burst your bubble; your body is seeking help. If you do not respond to your body's plea, your die-off, healing crisis or symptoms will get worse.

On October ninth, I had the colonoscopy done as I also dropped off a stool sample that had two worms in it. One of them was white and longer than a ruler, and the other one was half the size of the white one. My friend Donna worked that particular day, so after talking to the receptionist, I asked Donna to call the microbiology department and speak to the supervisor for me. In fact, Donna allowed me to chat with the supervisor.

"Hello."

"Hi."

"Hi, Sue this is Kelley. Donna is about to send a stool specimen down for me, and I want your techs to know that there are two parasites at the bottom of the container. As a previous tech, I know some med techs collect the specimen from the top and more than often the entire specimen isn't observed."

"When the specimen comes down, the tech remixes it."

'I understand that, but I'm asking you and them to take an extra step and go to the bottom of the container and get the worms from there. I have released over thirty worms, and I need to know what they are. I'm about to have a colonoscopy, and I don't want those worms missed. Is it okay if I write on a label, parasites or worms at the bottom of the container?"

"Sure, yes you can do that."

"Thank you, Sue, I appreciate you."

"You're welcome, and we will look for your specimen."

Donna wrote what I mentioned on the label and another sheet of paper in large print and stuck the paper in the bag. I had to be sure the techs would not miss those worms.

"Thank you so much, Donna. I appreciate you."

"You're welcome Kelley."

We hugged and said our goodbyes.

I went over to the Center for Care and Discovery and had the colonoscopy done. Before my procedure, I discussed my healing crisis with the nurse. She was amazed at the images of the worms and insisted that I take my cell phone into the procedure room to show the doctor. One of the other nurses started an IV on me and asked a question.

"Have you left the country within the last three to six months?"
"No, I have not left the country in the last three to six months or ever for that matter. Mainstream would have you think intestinal parasites are uncommon in America and that is far from the truth. These worms come from us eating the larvae of pork, beef, and fish. Infected animals and undercooking their meat leads to ingesting larvae. It is just that simple.
"How did you get them out of you?"
"I used turpentine and some other natural products. I also did enemas to flush them out of me."
"Wow. I'd like to do them."
"Well, all of this information will be in my book this coming January"
"We need the name of your book so we can buy it when you release it." Mary interrupted me.
"I will personally come over here after the book is published and bring it, Mary. You are the first person in this hospital to listen to me since this began."
"If you had seen me between August of last year and April of this year, you would think differently."
"Were you sick?"
"Very. My entire body was inflamed, burning; I couldn't sleep, or wear clothes."
"Did it itch?"
"Badly, sometimes so bad I cried like a baby. I was very miserable."
"Why didn't the doctors here give you anything?"
"They thought all this on my body was just a skin condition."
The nurse shook her and slightly frowned.

"What did you do?"

"I did a detox, cleaned my colon and changed the way I eat."

"What do you eat now?"

"I eat fruits and vegetables, chickpeas, some beans, red and black rice, quinoa and almonds. I avoid any foods that feed yeast or worms like blood, starch, and sugar and I drink a lot of water. I might eat some chicken maybe once or twice a month."

"How is your health?"

"It's better than ever now, I mean besides releasing these worms and yeast. I don't have hypothyroidism, high blood pressure or early stage heart disease anymore. I release forty-three pounds, and my skin has healed. What you see is just extra melanin or hyperpigmentation."

"I was going to ask how much weight you lost."

"I released a total of forty-three pounds. I weighed 178 pounds before I started healing my body."

How much do you weigh now? The male nurse interjected.

"I weigh 135 pounds."

"That is wonderful." Male nurse taps my hand as he proceeds to start my IV.

"My sister had parasites, but it didn't turn out that well for her. You look terrific. The nurse is on her way to get you and take you back for your procedure. Make sure you show those pics to the doctor." Mary was adamant about me showing those pictures to the doctor.

"Thank you and I will."

Both nurses left, and I was hauled off for my procedure. I made it to the procedure room and showed the doctor the images and videos of what I released from my body. After looking at the pictures, Dr. Mason mentioned them being tapeworms. As a little girl, I remember removing pinworms from my anus. I spoke to Sam in the Microbiology department, and he told me the material he examined was a very, very long mucus strand that looked similar to a tape worm. Sam also mentioned what I knew; that amount of mucus was very abnormal and that he was willing to test all material I released. That never happened.

The colonoscopy report revealed a diffuse area of moderate melanosis found in the entire colon and a few small diverticula in the sigmoid and descending colon. Biopsies were taken throughout the entire colon for histology. The examination was otherwise normal as no worms were seen. I wonder how and why? I mean that would be great if I released all of them. But, somehow I don't believe that to be true. Worms are known for migrating to other areas of the body, and I think that was Dr. Mason didn't see any worms. The whole purpose of the colonoscopy was to look for them. What's more, colonoscopies do not examine the small intestine.

The melanosis was something special to me as if you recall the beginning of this healing crisis, I was beet red and highly inflamed, however, since I've cleansed my colon, detoxed my body and changed my eating habits, my colon is no longer inflamed. Hallelujah!! So, what happened and why was my colon covered in dark spots. According to Miller-Keane (1999) melanosis is a condition characterized by dark pigmentary deposits throughout the colon. According to Dr. Mason, and medicinenet.com, melanosis is said to be caused by herbal enemas and laxatives that contain senna and cascara. I found that information to be interesting since I have not taken one herbal enema since I began treating myself. The only one I used was organic coffee and apple cider vinegar. After I ate that cheese and catfish, I did a lemon water enema and a garlic enema. So unless apple cider vinegar, lemons, and coffee, contain senna and cascara, I am not convinced that those enemas caused any pigmentation in my colon.

Here is my theory. The same way my skin was inflamed is the same way my colon looked before I started my natural healing. Did I have a colonoscopy before my healing? No, I did not. However, I had one in that past when I suffered from diarrhea, constipation, skin disorders, and inflammatory bowel disease and my colon was bright red. How do I know? I awoke during my past colonoscopy and asked the doctor if I could see my intestine. He turned the screen around, and my intestine was beet red. And from my experience in healthcare, red means inflammation or blood. So, I think that is enough information to conclude that my intestines were inflamed and after my natural treatment, the red color became dark or black just like my skin. Just because a doctor is a doctor, it does not mean what comes out of his mouth is correct.

My next appointment with Dr. Mason was set for December 11th and not much happened other than dialogue and an order for an X-Ray of my intestines that I have not scheduled yet. I've come to the conclusion that it doesn't matter what the doctors think or what test they run, I am the only one that can heal my body.

According to Miller-Keane, (1997) Diverticulitis is inflammation of the diverticula of the colon. Weaknesses of the muscles of the colon, sometimes produced by chronic constipation, leads to the formation of diverticula; small blind pouched that form in the lining and wall of the colon. Inflammation may occur as a result of collections of bacteria or other irritating agents trapped in the pouches; (Miller-Keane, 1997). Treatment consists of bed rest, cleansing enemas, a bland, low residue diet and drugs to reduce infection (Miller-Keane, 1997).

When I made it home, I looked at the video of the worms on my phone and googled images of tapeworms, and the photos were a splitting copy of what was in my videos. Adult tapeworms can measure more than fifty feet long and can survive as long as thirty years in a host. I have yet to find out what types of worms I have released. My test result was posted via My Chart and the ova and parasite results were as follows; No ova and parasites seen on concentration or special stain. Few leukocytes present. As I mentioned before, the O & P test is only about 50 to 60% accurate. What's more, the presence of leukocytes (White Blood Cells) means the presence of a pathogen. White blood cells come from the immune system. According to Mayo clinic, few or no leukocytes and many erythrocytes suggest the presence of Amebiasis (Entamoeba Histolytica, worm or parasite). Fecal leukocytes are rarely seen in diarrhea caused by other parasites or viruses (Mayo Clinic, 1995-2017).

In essence, the test result confirmed that there were worms present in my body and again, I have yet to discover what they are. In the meantime, Marc introduced me to another natural healing remedy that I was aware of, but never used, until now.

After experiencing all that I have and sharing it with you, I hope my story inspires you to take action and control of your health. I have spoken to numerous people who fear the absence of meat and starchy foods. I also know people who do not eat vegetables at all. However, these are the same people who complain about their weight and health. Fear is false evidence appearing real. Shift your focus to all the new foods you will have and not what you cannot have. What you put in your mouth is 85% health and wellness, exercise is 15% health and wellness, what you think is 100% health and wellness and what you feel is 1000% health and wellness. If you want health and wellness, it is time for you to transform your mindset as well as your eating habits. Transformation begins in your mind as patterns, behaviors, and practices live there. To shift your eating, you must change your thinking.

What doctors call symptoms are merely a sign of a toxic colon and a healing crisis as it all starts with what we ingest. So, I have one question for you. Are you ready to Detox or DIEt?

CHAPTER ELEVEN

Eat to Live

Eating clean was and still is the most challenging task. However, I do pretty well; consider I've eaten dirty for the last forty-five years. The hardest part for me was learning how to cook vegan dishes, clean foods, and different vegetables and just cooking real food period. Learning to season vegetables was a task for me as I stopped using seasoned salt and any other iodine salt-based seasons. I was accustomed to baking or boiling meat, like baked chicken, salmon or boiled turkey tails or necks. What's more, it was so easy to just cook a box of macaroni or some grits, or some rice-a-roni, or even drop some canned beans in a pot. I certainly enjoyed adding extra cheese to macaroni and then baking it until the cheese bubbled and slightly crisped. Man, do I miss cheese. But, I do not miss that constipation and death smelling farts. I started cooking at sixteen years young, and it was bacon and eggs. I burned the bacon, and in fact, I almost burned the kitchen down. Once I learned how to make breakfast, I started making dinner. My dinner consisted of a lot of canned foods, and processed meat, like chili, hotdog, salami, corned beef hash, peanut butter and jelly sandwiches and more of what I thought was food. It was so easy to cook processed foods and throw meat in the oven. I ate quite a bit of pork in my early twenties. I loved pork steak and Oscar Meyer hot dogs. The most I had to do was open a can, sprinkle some seasons, dump in flour, pour it in a pot or use the oven and that was easy. What's more, fast foods or restaurant foods were convenient and a quick way to go dirt surfing.

Over the past fifteen plus years, I rarely cooked or ate fried foods and certainly didn't eat pork or beef. I stopped sprinkling and eating sugar almost twenty years ago. I stopped drinking cow milk about ten years ago. However, I did still eat cheese as I loved pizza. Even if I ate pizza once a month, I had pepperoni on it. I mainly ate chicken, salmon, and turkey and was never good at frying chicken, so frying wasn't my thing at home. If I ate fried chicken, I bought it from J&J's, Wingz It Iz or Marianos. I also stopped at White Castles from time to time. And for whatever reason, I enjoyed farting the next day. At any rate, if I had to measure my eating habits on a scale of one to ten and ten being the worst, I would say it was about an eight. Some days I didn't eat meat at all. However, I didn't always add fruits and veggies to my meals either. Breakfast usually consisted of cinnamon toast crunch or honey nut cereals, oatmeal, grits with cheese, corned beef hash with poached eggs, a McDonald sausage, egg McMuffin sandwich, veggie omelettes, or a smoothie. So, I did eat real foods, however, not much. In fact, the only time I ate pork was when I ate McDonald's breakfast or pizza, and that was probably once or twice a month. Nonetheless, I didn't eat enough real foods like fruits and vegetable, and when I did eat them, they were GMO's.

GMO's are the most dangerous foods we can ingest. Sprayed with Round Up weed killer, a GMO is created by removing the DNA from a resistant seed (plant, crop) and inoculating it into a seed that is non-resistant. Once that gene has been placed into the non-resistant crop, it now resists herbicides and pesticides spray like Round Up and flourishes. The production is mass and a lot quicker than organic crop. Eating GMO's is eating Round-Up and according to Eco Watch, there are fifteen health problems linked to Monsanto's Round-Up. Read the article below.

15 Health Problems Linked to Monsanto's Roundup
(Eco Watch, Guest Contributor, 2015)
Monsanto invented the herbicide glyphosate and brought it to market under the trade name Roundup in 1974, after DDT was banned. But it wasn't until the late 1990s that the use of Roundup surged, thanks to Monsanto's ingenious marketing strategy. The strategy; genetically engineer seeds to grow food crops that could tolerate high doses of Roundup. With the introduction of these new GE seeds, farmers could now easily control weeds on their corn, soy, cotton, canola, sugar beets and alfalfa crops—crops that thrived while the weeds around them were wiped out by Roundup.

In the nearly 20 years of intensifying exposure, scientists have been documenting the health consequences of Roundup and glyphosate in our food, in the water we drink, in the air we breathe and where our children play. Eager to sell more of its flagship herbicide, Monsanto also encouraged farmers to use Roundup as a desiccant, to dry out all of their crops so they could harvest them faster. So Roundup is now routinely sprayed directly on a host of non-GMO crops, including wheat, barley, oats, canola, flax, peas, lentils, soybeans, dry beans and sugar cane.

Between 1996- 2011, the widespread use of Roundup Ready GMO crops increased herbicide use in the U.S. by 527 million pounds—even though Monsanto claimed its GMO crops would reduce pesticide and herbicide use. Monsanto has falsified data on Roundup's safety, and marketed it to parks departments and consumers as "environmentally friendly" and "biodegradable, to encourage its use it on roadsides, playgrounds, golf courses, schoolyards, lawns and home gardens. A French court ruled those marketing claims amounted to false advertising. In the nearly 20 years of intensifying exposure, scientists have been documenting the health consequences of Roundup and glyphosate in our food, in the water we drink, in the air we breathe and where our children play. They've found that people who are sick have higher levels of glyphosate in their bodies than healthy people. They've also found the following health problems which they attribute to exposure to Roundup and/or glyphosate:

ADHD*: In farming communities, there's a strong correlation between Roundup exposure and attention deficit disorder (ADHD), likely due to glyphosate's capacity to disrupt thyroid hormone functions.*

Alzheimer's disease: *In the lab, Roundup causes the same type of oxidative stress and neural cell death observed in Alzheimer's disease. And it affects CaMKII, an enzyme whose dysregulation has also been linked to the disease.*

147

Anencephaly (birth defect): *An investigation into neural tube defects among babies born to women living within 1,000 meters of pesticide applications showed an association for glyphosate with anencephaly, the absence of a major portion of the brain, skull and scalp that forms during embryonic development.*

Autism*: Glyphosate has a number of known biological effects that align with the known pathologies associated with autism. One of these parallels is the gut dysbiosis observed in autistic children and the toxicity of glyphosate to beneficial bacteria that suppress pathogenic bacteria, along with pathogenic bacteria's high resistance to glyphosate. In addition, glyphosate's capacity to promote aluminum accumulation in the brain may make it the principal cause of autism in the U.S.*

Birth defects: *Roundup and glyphosate can disrupt the Vitamin A (retinoic acid) signaling pathway, which is crucial for normal fetal development. The babies of women living within one kilometer of fields sprayed with glyphosate were more than twice as likely to have birth defects according to a study from Paraguay. Congenital defects quadrupled in the decade after Roundup Ready crops arrived in Chaco, a province in Argentina where glyphosate is used roughly eight to ten times more per acre than in the U.S. A study of one farming family in the U.S. documented elevated levels of glyphosate and birth defects in the children, including an imperforate anus, growth hormone deficiency, hypospadias (an abnormally placed urinary hole), a heart defect and a micro penis.*

Brain cancer: *In a study of children with brain cancer compared with healthy children, researchers found that if either parent had been exposed to Roundup during the two years before the child's birth, the chances of the child developing brain cancer doubled.*

Breast cancer: Glyphosate induces human breast cancer cells growth via estrogen receptors. The only long-term animal study of glyphosate exposure produced rats with mammary tumors and shortened life-spans.

Cancer: House-to-house surveys of 65,000 people in farming communities in Argentina where Roundup is used, known there as the fumigated towns, found cancer rates two to four times higher than the national average, with increases in breast, prostate and lung cancers. In a comparison of two villages, in the one where Roundup was sprayed, 31 percent of residents had a family member with cancer, while only 3 percent of residents in a ranching village without spraying had one. The high cancer rates among people exposed to Roundup likely stem from glyphosate's known capacity to induce DNA damage, which has been demonstrated in numerous lab tests.

Celiac disease and gluten intolerance: Fish exposed to glyphosate develop digestive problems that are reminiscent of celiac disease. There are parallels between the characteristics of celiac disease and the known effects of glyphosate. These include imbalances in gut bacteria, impairment in enzymes involved with detoxifying environmental toxins, mineral deficiencies and amino acid depletion.

Chronic kidney disease: Increases in the use of glyphosate may explain the recent surge in kidney failure among agricultural workers in Central America, Sri Lanka and India. Scientists have concluded, "Although glyphosate alone does not cause an epidemic of chronic kidney disease, it seems to have acquired the ability to destroy the renal tissues of thousands of farmers when it forms complexes with [hard water] and nephrotoxic metals."

Colitis: The toxicity of glyphosate to beneficial bacteria that suppress clostridia, along with clostridia's high resistance to glyphosate, could be a significant predisposing factor in the overgrowth of clostridia. Overgrowth of clostridia, specifically C. difficile, is a well-established causal factor in colitis.I was diagnosed with Colitis when I worked for the University of Chicago Hospital. I was about twenty-four or five years young. Treatment; Change your diet, nothing specifically.

Depression: Glyphosate disrupts chemical processes that impact the production of serotonin, an important neurotransmitter that regulates mood, appetite and sleep. Serotonin impairment has been linked to depression.

I suffered from depression during my early twenties and for two years.

Diabetes: Low levels of testosterone are a risk factor for Type 2 diabetes. Rats fed environmentally relevant doses of Roundup over a period of 30 days spanning the onset of puberty had reduced testosterone production sufficient to alter testicular cell morphology and to delay the onset of puberty.

Heart disease: Glyphosate can disrupt the body's enzymes, causing lysosomal dysfunction, a major factor in cardiovascular disease and heart failure.
In 2013, doctors at the University of Chicago Hospital diagnosed me with Coronary Atherosclerosis of the Native Coronary Artery. (Early Stage Heart Disease) Treatment: Eat more green veggies and lose weight.

Hypothyroidism: House-to-house surveys of 65,000 people in farming communities in Argentina where Roundup is used, known there as the fumigated towns, found higher rates of hypothyroidism.

In 2014, doctors at U of C diagnosed me with Hypothyroidism. Treatment: Levothyroxine.

Inflammatory Bowel Disease ("Leaky Gut Syndrome"): Glyphosate can induce severe tryptophan deficiency, which can lead to an extreme inflammatory bowel disease that severely impairs the ability to absorb nutrients through the gut, due to inflammation, bleeding and diarrhea.

It's interesting that "Leaky Gut Syndrome" is also considered Inflammatory Bowel Disease" I was diagnosed with IBS when I was about seventeen years old. No one ever mentioned that to me when I saw doctors at Cook County Hospital. Maybe the doctors had no idea or maybe they did. As I mentioned earlier, I remember having a colonoscopy at seventeen and I awoke during the procedure. I asked the doctor was it possible for me to see the screen. He repositioned the screen and I actually saw the inside of my colon. It was beet red and what the doctor considered highly inflamed. Again, the only treatment was for me to change my diet.

Liver disease: *Very low doses of Roundup can disrupt human liver cell function, according to a study published in Toxicology.*

Lou Gehrig's Disease (ALS): *Sulfate deficiency in the brain has been associated with Amyotrophic Lateral Sclerosis (ALS). Glyphosate disrupts sulfate transport from the gut to the liver, and may lead over time to severe sulfate deficiency throughout all the tissues, including the brain.*

Multiple Sclerosis (MS): *An increased incidence of inflammatory bowel disease (IBS) has been found in association with MS. Glyphosate may be a causal factor. The hypothesis is that glyphosate-induced IBS causes gut bacteria to leak into the vasculature, triggering an immune reaction and consequently an autoimmune disorder resulting in destruction of the myelin sheath.*

Non-Hodgkin lymphoma: *A systematic review and a series of meta-analyses of nearly three decades worth of epidemiologic research on the relationship between non-Hodgkin lymphoma (NHL) and occupational exposure to agricultural pesticides found that B cell lymphoma was positively associated with glyphosate.*

Parkinson's disease: The brain-damaging effects of herbicides have been recognized as the main environmental factor associated with neurodegenerative disorders, including Parkinson's disease. The onset of Parkinson's following exposure to glyphosate has been well documented and lab studies show that glyphosate induces the cell death characteristic of the disease.

Pregnancy problems (infertility, miscarriages, still births):
Glyphosate is toxic to human placental cells, which, scientists say, explains the pregnancy problems of agricultural workers exposed to the herbicide.

Obesity: An experiment involving the transfer of a strain of endotoxin-producing bacteria from the gut of an obese human to the guts of mice caused the mice to become obese. Since glyphosate induces a shift in gut bacteria towards endotoxin-producers, glyphosate exposure may contribute to obesity in this way.

Reproductive problems: Studies of laboratory animals have found that male rats exposed to high levels of glyphosate, either during prenatal or pubertal development, suffer from reproductive problems, including delayed puberty, decreased sperm production, and decreased testosterone production.

Respiratory illnesses: House-to-house surveys of 65,000 people in farming communities in Argentina where Roundup is used, known there as the fumigated towns, found higher rates of chronic respiratory illnesses (Eco Watch, Guest Contributor, 2015).
End Article

The exciting part of the article is that most of the dis-ease listed connects with parasites and yeast. What's more, I have experienced many of them besides colitis, and IBS, such as hypothyroidism, heart disease, obesity, and depression. You might think that there is a conflict with the articles I shared seeing as though all of them share variations in what's causing the healing crises we see in America. Well, the commonality is the gut. It doesn't matter if it's worms, yeast, mucoid plaque, GMO's or otherwise, all of the aforementioned wreaks havoc on the colon and therefore the entire body. As Dr. Anderson said, when the colon is sick, so are you. I shared all of those articles as I wanted you to become very familiar with what is killing us besides non-foods.

If this entire book doesn't make you want to become a breatharian, it should. Yes, live off air and light. Or at least create a sense of consciousness in what you put in your mouth today. The system has told us for so many years that we can eat meat, cheese, cow milk, bread, white sugar, and other bleached non-foods, GMO's and so much more and we believed them. The system has told us human intestinal parasites are not common in America. I beg to differ. I have not ever travelled outside of America so how did the worms that were inside me get there. The worms that were in my body probably came from ingesting the larvae of pork, fish and, or beef, food buffets, the dogs I grew up with, touching door knobs, eating off the ground and who knows where else. The point is I don't know how they got inside me other than it was definitely via my mouth and since I could remember and that was at 8 years old.

We have no idea whether our food is organic or not unless we grow it ourselves. However, we know we are sick, riddled with dis-ease and close to death. So, what is the gap between dis-ease and death? Let's look at the facts. GMO's, parasites (worms and candida), toxins and NON-FOODS; how do either of those make its way into our bodies? The gap between dis-ease and death is your mouth and what you put in it.

Today I choose to eat to live and not die. Dr. Sebi was right on point when he spoke on the alkaline diet, avoiding GMO's, eating live foods and at the cellular level. There are foods we should eat based on our blood types, as we should consume 80% alkaline foods and no more than 20% acid foods.

Today, my diet consists of eating with intention. By intention I mean, everything that goes in my mouth heals, empowers, and strengthens my body. Well, besides that glass of wine or chicken I might have from time to time. For the most part, my entire diet is 95% plant-based. I purposely make sure alkaline fruits and vegetable dominate my meals. What's more, I don't eat three times a day as I do not have too. I skip breakfast often. I know. You believe breakfast is the most important meal of the day and so you scramble your eggs, fry your sausage, chop your banana, and boil your oatmeal, pour your cereal and milk or whatever else you eat for breakfast. Well, I will have you know, the best meal you can have in the morning is hot water and freshly squeezed lemon juice. Water is a natural flush and gets the body moving in the morning as it aids in digestion. The most significant lemon water benefit is from the temperature of the water and not even the lemon. Drinking any water, (not tap water) or warm water, first thing in the morning can help flush the digestive system and rehydrate the body. I drink either room temperature, hot or warm water every morning and twenty-four ounces to be exact and of course, with a half of lemon as it contains Vitamin C and we know Vitamin C is good for the immune system as I eat clean.

So what does clean eating mean? Clean eating means to embrace a diet that includes whole foods. Whole foods are plant foods that are unrefined and unprocessed or refined and processed (no additives) as little as possible before consumption. Vegetable, fruits, nuts, seeds, legumes (beans) and grains are the example of whole foods. Some whole food examples are bananas, grapes, figs, mangoes, lemons, dandelion greens, and kale. Tomatoes, eggplant, 100% whole wheat pasta or bread, brown rice, olives, almonds, asparagus, mushrooms, kidney and lentil beans, chickpeas (garbanzo beans), navy, pinto and white beans, are also whole foods.

Eating clean also means to remove or cut-back on refined grains or those foods that lack the bran and germ. Some examples of processed grains are cornbread, corn tortillas, couscous, crackers, flour tortillas, grits, noodles, macaroni and pasta, pitas, pretzels, white bread, white rice, sandwich buns and rolls, and corn flakes. Removing the bran and germ gives the food a longer shelf life, but also eliminates iron, fiber, and some B vitamins. The white foods are bleached. In a nutshell, it's not good for the human body. I have yet to find pasta that interests me as I'm not a fan of wheat at all. However, I love quinoa, wild, red and black rice.

Another part of clean eating involves avoiding saturated fat, trans-fat, sugar and sugar-loaded drinks. Saturated fats are plainly put, bad fats and found in foods like pork, beef, milk, cream, cheese, and butter and a few more. Saturated fats have been linked to high cholesterol and cause heart disease. I would know. I weighed 165 pounds when doctors diagnosed me with high cholesterol and after that early stage heart disease. However, I no longer suffer from either as I no longer eat saturated fats.

According to a Mayo Clinic staff (2017), trans-fat or fatty acids are considered by many doctors to be the worst type of fat you can eat. Unlike other dietary fats, trans fat — also called trans-fatty acids — both raises your LDL ("bad") cholesterol and lowers your HDL ("good") cholesterol. A diet laded with trans-fat increases your risk of heart disease, the leading killer of men and women (Mayo Clinic staff, 2017).

Some meat and dairy products contain small amounts of naturally occurring trans-fat. But most trans-fat is formed through an industrial process that adds hydrogen to vegetable oil, which causes the oil to become solid at room temperature. This partially hydrogenated oil is less likely to spoil, so foods made with it have a longer shelf life. Some restaurants use partially hydrogenated vegetable oil in their deep fryers because it doesn't require frequent changing as do other oils (Mayo Clinic staff, 2017). Fried foods, doughnuts, cakes, cookies, crackers, pie crusts, biscuits, frozen pizza, margarine sticks and other spreads are loaded with trans-fats.

Sugar is death as we all know. And it's a great food for yeast to flourish and wreak havoc on you. Real sugar is brown, not white. Brown sugar undergoes the refining process to remove the molasses and giving it the white color. According to Appleton and Jacobs (2015), there are 141 ways sugar destroys your health.

Clean eating also involves removing pesticides, herbicides (Round-Up) additives, and preservatives, chemically charged foods from your diet. How do you do this? Read your labels and have a pair of readers (glasses) in your purse or pocket as I guarantee you will not be able to read the font as it will be a four. Stop adding white salt, sugar and seasoned salt to your food; those are chemicals. Stick with herbs like garlic, oregano, thyme, basil, turmeric, cayenne, cinnamon, cilantro, coriander, chives, ginger, curry, bay leaves, chili powder, dill weed, Himalayan salt, rosemary and nutritional yeast. Not only do these spices add flavor to your food, but they are great for you. And if I must add, parasites do not like, garlic, cayenne, or onions. There are plenty of spices and herbs that spruce up your food; you just have to be willing to buy and try them. I am still learning.

Real food comes from the earth, not the laboratory, the plant or the factory. After removing all of the foods above from your diet, you're probably wondering, what is left to eat? There is plenty. The question you should ask is how do you cook or prepare them? What types of meals do I create with fruits, veggies, nuts, beans, seeds and gluten and starch free grains? I will tell you. But, not before I share my favorite vegan dish. The best live food or vegan dish I have had thus far was prepared by Living Food Chef, Regina Thomas Dillard from Inner + Sanctum Wellness. Regina prepared vegan lasagna for my mastermind group, and I was highly impressed. The lasagna was so good I have to share the recipe with you as Regina permitted.

Raw Lasagna
Yield: 2-3 Servings
- 1-2 Zucchini, thinly sliced lengthwise

Nut Cheese
- 1 cup of Macadamia Nuts
- 1 cup of Cashews, soaked
- 2 Tbsp. Nama Shoyu Soy Sauce
- 2 Tbsp. Lemon Juice
- 2 Garlic Gloves, minced
- 1 Tbsp. each, Parsley, Chives

Tomato Sauce
- 1 Ripe tomato, seeded and chopped
- 1/2 cup of sun-dried tomatoes
- 1/2 red bell pepper
- 2 Tbsp. Extra Virgin Olive Oil
- 3 Basil Leaves
- 1 tsp dried Oregano
- 1/2 tsp. Garlic, minced
- 2 Medjool Dates, pitted

Basil Pesto
- 1 cup of Basil Leaves, tightly packed
- ½ cup of Raw Pistachios
- 1 tbsp. lemon juice
- 2 cup Spinach
- 2 tsp olive oil
- 1/2 tsp salt

Marinated Spinach
- 2 cups of Spinach
- 1 tsp Olive Oil
- 1/4 tsp Sea Salt

DIRECTIONS:
Prep Instruction:

With a mandolin, thinly slice zucchini and place in bowl. (This will mimic lasagna pasta). Drizzle with olive and salt   Set aside.

Cheese

Process all ingredients in food processor until smooth. Transfer to bowl and refrigerate.

Tomato Sauce
Process in a food processor until smooth

Pesto
Process all ingredients until combined. Do not over process.
Spinach
Place all ingredients in a bowl to marinate for 1 hour

To Assemble:
- Place zucchini strips on bottom of dish to serve as base.
- Spoon a thin layer of cheese on top of zucchini, followed by marinated spinach, tomato sauce, and then pesto on top.
- Repeat this process, starting with zucchini.
- Place dish in refrigerator a minimum of 4 hours to firm up.
- Use serrated knife to cut into individual portions.
- Garnish with a sprig of basil.

When I tell you that was the best vegan lasagna I have ever had, trust me, you will feel the same way. So go ahead and make it for yourself.

At any rate, learning to cook real food was like being a newborn in the kitchen. I learned to make raw, vegan tacos, and pasta, avocado sauce, hummus, a salad to die for, salad dressing using olive oil, lemons, and spices, eggplant, and cauliflower dishes, hearty soups, vegan chili, rutabaga chips, rice dishes, bread and a whole lot more. I had never even heard of black or red rice. I also introduced myself to different greens like chard and dandelion greens, bok choy (Chinese cabbage), and I taught myself to make a delicious quinoa and kale dish. So, you see, everything is about deprogramming, reconditioning and taking time to take care of you. You can do it. It may be complicated or confusing in the beginning, but a part of loving you is nurturing and nourishing your body. Health is your relationship with your body. Apparently, I had a horrible relationship with my body, but, keyword, had. I am delighted to say those days are over.

I screwed up several dishes and some days I wanted just to buy some chicken and pop it in the oven. Some days I wanted to order out and go back to my old ways. That was so much easier. What this comes down to is laziness, conditioning, resisting change and unwillingness to learn. You have to be open to unlearning, relearning and learning again. Everything you learned about eating was a lie, and some of us are aware of that, but we instead satisfy our tongues and addictions than feed our bodies what it needs to live. And I'm not harsh as that was me. I was so controlled or bonded by cheese; I had to have and daily. Did you know there is a chemical in cheese that is more addictive than heroin (What the Health? (Netflix Movie). You could not pay me to eat that snot today as that's all it is, cow mucus or snot. What's more, while we think our food taste "good," your non-foods are injected with a chemical that gives it a "good" taste. I don't see pork or beef tasting good. It is the chemical that gives it the taste.

Some of us call it celebrating or "eating good," when we have a T-bone or sirloin steak. How is that good eating when that dead beef is going to hang out in your colon and wreak havoc on you? I guess you saw that in a commercial as I did and believed you were doing something when you ingested $40 worth of death or dead energy. What's more, you are eating all of the emotions that cow, pig, chicken, turkey, and fish felt upon slaughtering. How is a steak made for starters? How is the meat held together and how does the pink color maintain even after death. You all know flesh decomposes after death. So, what are we eating? We are eating animal blood that which is death. What is salami? What is a hotdog? What is a polish? What is rice-a-roni? What is cheese? What are powdered potatoes? What are you eating? What was I eating? The only people who know the answers to those questions are the laboratory scientist who made the non-foods. But know this, real foods come from the ground and don't kill you. Real foods is live energy .Meat is dead energy. Stop feeding your live body dead energy as eventually, dead is exactly where you will be.

Are you okay with knowing you are killing yourself? The food scientist spends hours in the lab making non-foods into something we call food so they can maintain their elite lifestyles. But our lifestyles consist of slow death. Why can't we spend time in the kitchen learning how to feed our bodies and eat to live? Well, Americans are programmed to work and eat processed and fast food. We are not trained to take care of ourselves as we are taught to "take care" of others, and that includes helping millionaires become billionaires. We awake in the morning, stop at a fast food restaurant for breakfast, go to work (take care of someone else) and wear ourselves out. We go to lunch at another fast food restaurant and then go back to work. Then we get off and stop at another fast food restaurant. Rarely do we go to the gym after eating all the dead energy, we go to sleep and repeat the vicious cycle of a slow death the next day. It is time for us to eat to live, not live to eat or eat to die. What's more, instead of preparing our foods, like cleaning vegetables, chopping, soaking, dehydrating, or seasoning them, we buy it already processed, packed and ready to cook or eat. Is it laziness or it conditioning? I think it's a combination of both. After being conditioned for so long by your parents or whoever raised you, you become stuck in your eating and cooking patterns and behaviors as laziness sets in and you don't want to learn. So, maybe it's a bit of brain laziness as well.

I have learned so much about real food since Mr. Parasite and Ms. Yeast showed up in my life. Life is good, and pain is power. One of the benefits I appreciate about eating clean is there is no such thing as being sleepy after eating. Some of us think that is normal; however, that is far from the truth. The reason people become sleepy after eating is that we consume dead energy like meat, pasta, and starchy carbohydrates. It takes so much energy or blood oxygen to digest meat and starch that the body becomes tired. Eating clean gives you strength.

What's more, I feel great after eating. The last time I felt exhausted after eating was last year, and I don't remember the exact time.

The most important benefits of eating whole and clean are receiving the full amount of vitamins, minerals, fiber, healthy fats, carbohydrates, and proteins. The combination of those creates a healthy body as they work to prevent dis-ease. Lastly, you create longevity, wholesome and correctly functioning organs, brain clarity, more energy, and so much more.

Your body desires nutrition, and once the body has it, you will feel full. Nutrition moves through the body and feeds our cells and rapidly as it is light energy. However, when you ingest foods like burgers, Italian beef, pizza, fries, hot dogs, white rice, cereal and any other processed food, you eat more because the body doesn't recognize any nutrition. Therefore, you eat more, then overeat, gain weight and create disease. Feed your body, not your fat cells was a phrase I learned in school for Health Information Management. Today, that phrase should be feed your body, not worms and yeast.

Ninety-nine percent of the American non-food diet feed parasites, such as yeast and worms. We have to be diligent in learning how to eat again. It wasn't easy for me, as my creations do not always turn out good, but I do try, and we all know, practice makes perfect. I learned a lot about foods at the Whole Foods store in Orland Park, Illinois.

There are two stores that I predominately shop for organic foods, Whole Foods and Mariano's. Most grocery stores have become aware of people shifting to whole foods and have created a natural section in their stores. Jewels and Aldi's have organic products. The whole foods store in Orland Park is my absolute favorite and not just because of the food and whole body department, but because the people are extraordinarily kind. There was one gentleman in particular who expressed just how kind and warm humans can be. Every month or every two weeks,

I shopped at the Whole Foods for my supplements and foods. Bill, an employee, was always so willing to help me. Even when my skin was in the worst condition, Bill never frowned upon me. He found every product I needed, compared a few and told me what he thought was best. I had a list every time I came in and Bill always said, just give me the list as I followed him around in the whole body department. He was never impatient or afraid to stand next to me. In fact, every employee I presented myself to was very kind, willing to help and even if that meant stepping out of their department. But, Bill was my favorite and because of Bill, I felt comfortable walking around in the store with my damaged skin. I thanked him one day during my usual trip.

"Hey Bill."

"Hey, how are you? Bill was always so enthusiastic and had a great smile.

"Do you recall when I first came in here last year seeking supplements to help my skin condition?" Bill was stocking the freezers.

"Yeah, I do" Bill stepped off of the stool he was on to give me his full attention.

"Well, I finally figured out what it was. Every diagnosis the doctors told me was wrong. I have parasites in my body and an overgrowth of yeast. When they die, they release over eighty toxins in my body."

"Wow. Oh my God honey. I'm so sorry this is happening to you."

"Well, it's okay. I finally have control, and now I can heal my body completely. But I wanted to thank you for being so kind to me. You never judged me, and you were always willing to help me." My eyes filled with tears. "You never frowned upon me and behaved as if you didn't want to stand next to me. I felt so comfortable with you, and I just want to say thank you so much. You don't know how much you helped me."

"Oh wow. I'm so happy to hear that. I'm leaving the store in two weeks."

"Oh wow. I'm going to miss you." I wiped my tears as they flowed from down my face.

"Thank you, and this makes me feel good too. I've worked two jobs, and I need more time for my family. So, I'm leaving for a better paying job and that way I only have to work one."

"I'm happy things are working out for you. Your wife is very blessed to have you. You have such a compassionate heart."

"Thank you, but I'm blessed to have her. She's up front. She works here too. She's the small brunette at the front register."

"Oh wow. I'm going to go and say hi to her. Well, I don't want to hold you up any longer, so again, thank you so much for helping me and never judging me. I am so grateful to you."

Bill and I hugged, and I went on my way.

Thank you again, Bill, for your compassion, kindness, and willingness to help me. I will never forget you.

Just as I am grateful for Bill, I am even more thankful for the Whole Foods store. I took anywhere from 10 to 15 supplements per day, and whole foods stocked every one of them. Well, except a few teas I needed, but that was okay as Bill told me which store to go to find any products that they might not have. I learned about coconut chips, grain free tortillas, cassava taco shells, dandelion greens, curry paste as I don't eat tomato paste, organic lipstick, lotion, soap and so much more. I spend anywhere from one to three hours in the whole foods store. And I learned how to shop there without breaking the bank. The first time I went to the whole foods store (2014) I spent over $400 and had about seven bags. You're probably wondering what was in those seven bags. I'm still trying to figure it out today. However, I have shopping and saving at whole foods down to a science. Let's not talk about the restaurant section, my goodness that foods taste so fresh. My son and husband love the Larry Killer deli sandwich, and I must agree that sandwich is bomb-diggity. They even have vegan pizza, and it's delicious. Sometimes, I walk through the store and just sample foods before shopping for anything. Another great thing about the whole foods in Orland Park is that if you have never tasted the product, they have a "try it on us" deal, and you don't have to pay for it. Recently, I learned the "try it in us" deal has ended. Now, that does not include every item as I believe it is based on price and depends on the product. At any rate, I have never experienced that in any store. I love the whole foods store and recommend their food, service, and products to anyone. If you haven't shopped at the Whole Foods store, you need to and if you need help, reach out to me. As a Coach, I would be more than happy to take you on your first trip. Trust me, once you go in, coming out will be challenging as learning about foods is good for the body.

The employees are very knowledgeable, and the labels are legible. Many of the employees know me as I am a regular customer who always asks questions. The list goes on. So, when you shop at the whole foods, you don't have to be afraid, just shop, feel good and create optimal health. In essence, the Whole Foods store played an enormous role in healing my body and creating optimal health. In fact, the whole foods store is another aspect of raising my vibrations.

CHAPTER TWELVE

Illness Raises Your Vibrations

Since Ms. Yeast and Mr. Parasite presented themselves, I have thoroughly raised my vibrations or energy. Most of us get caught up in the illness or negative energy and never witness the lesson and blessing. What's more, we refuse to see that we created the disease or dis-ease. I tried to quit smoking over a hundred times and always started back. I attempted to release the excess weight, but either I gained it back or never released it. I wanted to release the desire for hard liquor and wine. I also desired a vegan or vegetarian lifestyle. I wanted my body to heal and release the high blood pressure, high cholesterol, hypothyroidism, joint pain and other ailments. I tried, but maybe not hard enough.

Dis-ease is not intended for our demise as everything we experience in life is for our highest good. However, we have been taught to behave like victims and relinquish our power over to the system. I asked for exactly what I received, pain and all. What's more, dis-ease is a healing crisis as it is your body's way of telling you to change your lifestyle and heal. A healing crisis does not mean your life is over, nor does it mean run to the doctor. It means stop doing the things you are doing and allow and assist your body in healing. Do you think I would be in the happy and healed space I am in if I had kept smoking, drinking, eating meat, and processed foods? I highly doubt as my body would've failed. You have to love, nourish and give your body what it needs, not respond to cravings and feed it garbage. Your body is always healing as it is ready, but when you continually add unhealthy products, you are destined to create a healing crisis.

If you are in a healing crisis, there are a few things you must do to raise your vibration and maintain higher frequencies. The list below describes the process I used to heal my emotional and mental body.

1. Accept Your Part in the Creation of the Healing Crisis

Dis-ease isn't hereditary as there are causes and cures for all dis-ease or healing crises. Accept your part in its creation as you are a co-creator. You did it so don't blame any person in your life for the amount of stress or experiences you have. Don't blame the food as you opened your mouth and ate it. Don't blame the system as there is more than enough information in the world and we all have access to it. The best University one can ever attend if YouTube University.

2. Remove All Things that No Longer Serve You a Purpose

The commonality for creating all disease is what we ingest or put into our bodies. So, why are you still ingesting or inhaling foods or toxins that assist in the breakdown of your body? Meat, processed foods, nicotine, drugs, alcohol, tap water and anything else that you know you should not have needs to be removed.

3. Accountability for Thoughts, Emotions, and Behaviors

Stop blaming and take your power back. If you respect the fact that your thoughts are yours and are the source of creation, then you can respectfully acknowledge them and stop amplifying unhealthy thoughts with the corresponding emotion. The more you blame others, the more you give your power away. Own your feelings and do the work to release them. Be honest about your feelings whether they are fear, jealousy, anger, sadness, embarrassment or guilt. Be honest and release them. Emotions cause dis-ease. In fact, a disease is highly based on thought-forms as your emotions amplify it and the behavior creates it. You are the reason you are in the space you are in, not your mother, father, boyfriend, girlfriend, job or otherwise. Blaming leads to lack of growth, in all areas.

4. Gratitude

Gratitude is the attitude. If you are not grateful for what you have and always complain about what you don't have, you will receive more to complain about. You have to be mindful of what you have in front of you as gratitude attracts more gratitude. If you are not grateful for you small apartment, why would you be grateful for your large home? They are both shelter yet one is bigger than the other. Always be grateful for everything and more will present itself. Stop whining and complaining and name five things you are grateful for daily.

5. Forgive

For all dis-ease, there is an unhealthy thought and emotion stuck in your mind and heart. That belief and feeling stem from some old childhood or deep-rooted pan that you refuse to accept and let go. Therefore you must learn the process of forgiveness as it has nothing to do with anyone but you. Forgiveness is about releasing the anger, bitterness, and resentment you're harboring so you can free yourself. Listed below are my five steps to forgiveness.

a. Grieve

Release the pain via tears, talking and writing. Harboring unhealthy energy destroys your body. In fact, guilt and shame create cancer, and you wonder why I am shameless and live a guilt-free life. Tears are a sign of life, and it was the first thing you did at birth. If you refuse to feel, you can't cry, meaning you are a dead man walking. Healing requires feeling. Have your five minutes of self-pity and move forward.

Every tear shed is a sign of strength and freedom to come.

b. Compassion

Compassion is just as about you as forgiveness is. However, compassion is a deep feeling of empathy or sadness for someone who suffers as hurt people hurt people and you want them to heal. Even the person that murders or robs and rape deserves compassion as they suffer. For people to stop projecting pain onto other people, they must recover. It is essential to have compassion for others as if you don't have it for others; you won't have it for self. Everything starts with you.

c. **Acceptance**

What happened; has happened and will not change. Accept the fact that you were hurt and scars are present. Accept the fact that you may have allowed continuous pain in your life. Therefore you created it. More than often we have to accept things that we don't want to accept, and that doesn't mean, the experience was "okay," however, it does suggest, you will be okay, and the experience is not going anywhere. You may also have to accept the fact that you abused yourself or maybe you disrespected your body over and over again and knew your ill will. Be okay with that, have compassion for you and move forward.

d. **Accountability**

No one is responsible for you but you. Neither the doctors nor the pastor is responsible for you. Your parents may have raised you in dysfunction, but you are responsible for staying there and experiencing whatever you experience today. Stop blaming; who cares if you learned how to eat poorly as a child? That is neither here nor there as what matters is you are accountable for everything in your life today.

e. **Learn From It - Find Something Positive**

One of the critical elements of forgiveness is to learn from the painful experience. There is a lesson in everything we experience. It doesn't matter how harmful, malicious or callous; there is a lesson. To learn from hurt is to gain strength. To learn from pain is to gain knowledge. To learn from harm represent growth and maturity. Find something positive as there is always one. Did you learn something about yourself during this experience? Did it make you a better person? Learn from all experiences, as no experience is a bad experience if you get the lesson. They are all blessings.

When I talk about unhealthy energy, low vibrations or low frequencies, I speak to the following emotions (energy in motion); shame, guilt, apathy, grief, desire, pride, and fear.

The following levels and explanations of energy or emotions are from Power vs. Force by Dr. David Hawkins (2012).

When people are blamed for things, and that experience is a negative one, he or she might feel guilty. Recall in my first book, Perfectly Planned; I was blamed for being sexually molested, and the guilt practically killed my person. Having guilt leads to psychosomatic diseases, being accident prone or suicidal behavior. Guilt can also provoke rage or murder (Hawkins, 2012). Shame is expressed after humiliation and leads to hanging your head low, wishing you were invisible and prone to physical illness (Hawkins 2012). So many times after I drank or smoked a cigarette I felt so much shame as I knew both were deteriorating my health. Apathy is provoked by despair and characterized by poverty, hopelessness, neediness, victim mindset, and or suicide (Hawkins 2012). At one point, I felt like I lost control of my health as I lost interest in eating to live. According to Hawkins (2012), grief is provoked by regret and characterized by a certain level of sadness, loss or dependency. Those who live at this level live a consistent life of anxiety and depression. When one lives in fear, the viewpoint of the world looks dangerous and full of traps and threats. Fear limits the growth of the personality and may take any form (Hawkins, 2012). Directly after the inflammation subsided, I worried about what people would think of my skin. Today, I have no cares about what people think of me as it is none of my business.

When one expresses desire, it represents craving and can also be at the level of addiction. Desire is directly related to accumulation and greed (Hawkins, 2012). Wants can start us on the road to achievement as they can also assist us in performance and become a springboard of higher levels of awareness (Hawkins, 2012. I had a strong desire for cigarettes and alcohol, and the cigarettes were an addiction, though, the liquor was not, but, my body desired it to the point of destroying my body.

Pride in contrast to the lower energy fields, people feel positive as they reach this level. However, Pride feels good only in comparison to the lower levels (Hawkins, 2012). For example, you failed your midterm exam, and after the retake, you scored a one hundred percent. Pride is defensive and vulnerable because it's dependent upon external conditions, without which can suddenly revert to a lower level. Inflated ego fuels pride, hence the downside of pride is arrogance and denial. These characteristics block growth (Hawkins, 2012).

Anger expresses itself most often as resentment and revenge and is, therefore, volatile and dangerous (Hawkins, 2012). Since anger stems from frustrated wants, the energy field is below it. Frustration results from exaggerating the importance of desires. Anger leads easily to hatred, which has an erosion effect on all areas of a person's life (Hawkins, 2012). I was angry at the doctors for misdiagnosing me. However, my anger came from wanting to know what happened inside my body and rightfully so. The power was, is and always will be inside me. Deep inside I was angry because I lost control of my health.

Those emotions are considered low vibration as they lower our mood, energy, mindset, and person as a whole. When we look at high vibrations, we look at emotions like neutrality, consciousness, acceptance, reason, joy, peace and enlightenment (Hawkins, 2012). Energy gets very positive as we get to this level.

Neutral conditions allow for flexibility and nonjudgmental, realistic appraisal of problems (Hawkins, 2012). To be neutral means to be relatively unattached to outcomes; not getting one's way is no longer experienced as defeating, frightening or frustrating (Hawkins, 2012). People at this level are easy to get along with and safe to be around and associate with because they are not interested in conflict, competition or guilt. These people are comfortable and relatively undisturbed emotionally. This attitude is nonjudgmental and doesn't lead to any need to control other people's behavior (Hawkins, 2012).

Willingness is a level of consciousness perceived as a gateway to the higher levels. At the neutral level, jobs are done adequately, but at the level of willingness, work is done well, and success in all endeavors is obvious (Hawkins, 2012). Growth is rapid here; these are people chosen for advancement. At this level, people become genuinely friendly and social and economic success seems to follow automatically. People here are helpful to others and contribute to the good of society (Hawkins, 2012). They're also willing to face internal issues and don't have learning blocks. With their capacity to bounce back from adversity and learn from experience, they tend to become self-correcting. Having let go of pride, they're willing to look at their defects and learn from others (Hawkins, 2012).

At the acceptance level, a major transformation takes place, with the understanding that one is oneself the source and creator of the experience of one's life (Hawkins, 2012). At the Acceptance stage, nothing "out there" can make one happy, and love isn't something that's given or taken away by another but created from inside. Acceptance allows engagement in life on life's terms, without trying to make it conform to an agenda (Hawkins, 2012). The individual at this level isn't interested in determining right or wrong but instead is dedicated to resolving issues and finding out what to do about problems (Hawkins, 2012).

Reason is the level when intelligence and rationality rise to the forefront when the emotionalism of the lower levels is transcended (Hawkins, 2012). This is the level of science, medicine, and of generally increased capacity for conceptualization and comprehension. Knowledge and education here are sought as capital (Hawkins, 2012).

Love is unconditional, unchanging, and permanent. It doesn't fluctuate – its source isn't dependent on external factors (Hawkins, 2012). Loving is a state of being. It's a forgiving, nurturing, and supportive way of relating to the world. Love isn't intellectual and doesn't proceed from the mind; (Hawkins, 2012). Love emanates from the heart. Only 0.4% of the world's population ever reaches this level of evolution of consciousness (Hawkins, 2012).

As love becomes more and more unconditional, one experiences inner joy. Joy arises from each moment of existence, rather than from any other source (Hawkins, 2012). A capacity for enormous patience and the persistence of a positive attitude in the face of prolonged adversity is characteristic of this energy field; the hallmark of this state is compassion. People who have attained this level have a notable effect on others (Hawkins, 2012). They're capable of a prolonged, open gaze, which induces a state of love and peace. The world one sees is illuminated by the exquisite beauty and perfection of creation. Everything happens effortlessly and by synchronicity (Hawkins, 2012).

Peace associates with the experience designated by such terms as transcendence, self-realization, and God-consciousness. It's extremely rare, attained by only 1 in 10 million people (Hawkins, 2012). When one obtains peace, the distinction between subject and object disappears, and there's no specific focal point of perception. This astonishing revelation takes place non-rationally so that there is an infinite silence of mind, which has stopped conceptualizing (Hawkins, 2012). The observer and the thing that is witnessed takes on the same identity; the observer dissolves into the landscape and becomes equally the observed (Hawkins, 2012).

Enlightenment is the level of the Great Ones of history which originated the spiritual patterns that countless people have followed throughout the ages (Hawkins, 2012). Enlightenment is the level of inspiration; these beings set in place attractor energy fields that influence all of the mankind. At this level there is no longer the experience of an individual personal self-separate from others; instead, there is an identification of self with consciousness and divinity (Hawkins, 2012). Enlightenment is the peak of the evolutionary consciousness in the human realm. At this level there is no longer any identification with the physical body as "me," and therefore, its fate is of no concern (Hawkins,

2012). The body is merely a tool of consciousness through the intervention of mind; its prime value is that of communication, and this level is of non-duality, or complete Oneness (Hawkins, 2012)

So, how did this healing crisis raise my mental, emotional, physical and soul vibrations? In more ways than I ever imagined. After thirty-two years of smoking cigarettes, I no longer smoke cigarettes. I never had enough faith in myself to quit smoking as I didn't understand my internal powers. I have tried so many times to quit smoking and started back each time. I was afraid of the weight gain as I made an excuse after excuse. I even went as far as to say, Salem Lights 100 was not as bad a Newport's; cognitive dissonance. My desire or addiction to nicotine was compelling; however, my health outweighed that craving. With that, I became the most important thing to me.

After twenty-five years of drinking and abusing alcohol, I no longer drink alcohol. Alcohol was my way of celebrating, partying, hanging with friends or just socializing. Eventually, it became a habit as my body desired it more than often. During my healing crisis, I realized my body was a gift from the Universe, and I must respect, love and not abuse it. I did not want to cause my body any more pain or feed it any more toxins as I had enough. My body has been very patient with me, and it was time for me to finally love and honor my body as I had not before. I decided to release the desire for alcohol, and today I am alcohol-free. I have had a couple of glasses of wine; however, I choose to live a sober life. In essence, Mr. Worm and Ms. Yeast taught me how to love my body and release the desire for alcohol, however, I might have a glass of wine from time to time. What's more, I learned how to socialize without alcohol and simply be present to the moment with my husband, friends, and family. I no longer need anything but my free and sober mind.

Mentally speaking, and understanding how thoughts initiate the process of creations, I pay close attention to mine. I know before this healing crisis, I thought I was a horrible person for not being able to care for my son and help my husband. I also thought I was worthless and felt awful about my person. Today, regardless of the decisions I make, I always know that I am going in the best direction for me. With that understanding, I will no longer think unkind thoughts of myself. I am divine and every idea I think leads to an emotion that amplifies the idea and following that is the creation. I create wisely in my find first. I choose loving and joyous thoughts as I create a safe, loving and joyous world. I am safe and free. I am health, wealth and success.

Emotionally speaking, I understand that emotions and disease go hand in hand and with that knowledge, I now involve myself in healthy emotions. If any experience arises that in any other case, I would react in fear and anger, today I choose to respond in love and compassion. If I feel any negative emotions, I release them and move away from them. I do not avoid or lie to myself. I practice empathy and forgiving others. What's more, I see people through my soul's eyes instead of my ego eyes.

I am also emotionally intelligent and aware of where my emotions originate as I am also accountable for them. That paradigm makes a huge difference. As long as I understand that I am responsible for what and how I feel, I can just acknowledge, shift, learn and move forward. Mr. Parasite and Ms. Yeast raised my emotional vibrations in a mighty fine way. I am alive to the joys of living. I deserve and accept the very best in life. I love and approve of myself.

Physically speaking, I released forty-three pounds of waste. I was at an all-time high of 178 pounds as my stomach hung and touched my thighs. I know some people may say, you were thick or you carried the weight well. Well, I'd like to know how does one carry waste well. The forty-four pounds I released was waste, toxins, excess water, garbage, feces and other crap that slowly killed me. I didn't realize just how huge I was until I looked at an old picture of me (See the back of the book). Again, Mr. Parasite and Ms. Yeast showed up and showed out and for my benefit. Sure, there was a lot of pain and suffering. However, I now weigh 134 pounds and feel like I did when I was in my twenties.

Let's talk about my lab values before my detox and cleanse. I had a wellness check on October 18, 2017, and compared to last year's results. Last year in October, my total cholesterol was 218. The normal range is 125 - 199. Today, my total cholesterol is 195. My LDL cholesterol was 145. The normal range is less than 130. Today my LDL is 119. My body mass index or BMI was 31.3, and today it is 24.7. According to the European standard, the normal range for someone my height is 18.5 – 24.9. My blood pressure was 137/86, and today it is 108/65. Although it wasn't abnormal October 2016, by the time February 2017 approached, my BP held steady at 150/ 100. Three consecutive visits to the doctor's office with a high blood pressure is a diagnosis of hypertension. What's more, my waist circumference was a 36, and today it is 28. I lost 8 inches off my waste. My eyes or sclera is no longer yellow as they have cleared and my fingernails develop rapidly. Now that is phenomenal. Lastly, my thyroid, as I mentioned, I was diagnosed with hypothyroidism in July of 2014. My thyrotropin or TSH was slightly high (4.91) as the range is 0.30 – 1.00 and according to doctors that indicated an underacting thyroid. I took levothyroxine daily for the last three years and in May of 2017; I decided to stop and focus on my Spiritual Detox. In July 2017, I had my blood drawn, and my thyrotropin was 8.56 (very high). However, my T3 and T4 were standard. On October 18, 2017, my thyrotropin was 4.76, and both the T3 and T4 are normal. How cool is that? I healed my thyroid. I can guarantee before January 2017 my TSH will be within the European standard range. I am excited as in my head, I have healed my thyroid with food, detoxing and cleansing my body.

What does all that mean? I created optimal health. What's more, the mere fact that I released the waste, cleansed my colon detoxed my body and all my values became normal that tells me that health is in what we eat as well as what we harbor in our gut (colon). My journey describes taking control of your health and not relying on doctors to prescribe pills for healing. Healing starts with you. I lovingly take back my power and eliminate all interference.

Soulfully speaking, I've done a lot of work in this lifetime, both physical and soul. The physical work I've done aligns with my soul's work. It is no wonder; I chose healthcare as my physical body suffered from dis-ease for over three decades. What's more, my soul's work I do today aligns with my emotional and mental being. You don't believe me becoming an author, speaker and coach are coincidental. It's all divine and aligned.

My mental, emotional, physical and soul being needed profound healing so every path I took, every incident I experienced, every job I worked, every client I coached, every presentation I spoke and every book I wrote, was FOR me first. My soul has aligned with the Universe since birth, but my person was resistant and ignorant. And that is okay. It took ignorance, resistance, and dis-ease to raise my vibrations and today, I walk in purpose and on purpose.

I am at peace with it all as when the time comes for this physical body to transition; I know my soul will return. But this time, in a much higher vibration. My soul's work has raised my vibrations in leaps and bounds, and now I share it all with you to help you transform and reach a level of neutrality, love, peace, joy, acceptance, and maybe even enlightenment.

I am enlightened. I am joy. I am light. I am spirit. I am love.

On October 19, 2017, I visited the University of Chicago hospital one last time as I took seven small jars of worms, mucus, and yeast. One of the nurses told me I could come in and see an urgent care physician and bring the worms in. My chief goal was to have the worms identified. It was no doubt that I released worms, but my ego wanted to know what they were. Dr. Alex wasn't interested in my reality or sending the worms down for testing.

"Hi Mrs. Porter-Turner, my resident explained to me a few things that you would like to have done, so I'd like to hear it from you."

"Well, last August, I was diagnosed with Psoriasis, Pityriasis Rosacea, and Lichen Planus. I learned that all three of those diagnoses were wrong. I decided to heal myself holistically. I used natural herbs, and supplements as well as enemas. My skin is a lot better as I feel great. I've released 43 pounds as well as a lot of worms, candida yeast, and mucus. I have several worms and other foreign objects in those jars. I would like them tested. I would also like to have an MRI or another scan to identify where the worms hide in my body. The colonoscopy doesn't check the small intestine so I want to know if we can move forward with some different procedures."

"Well, first, I think you irritated the lining of your intestine with what you have done."

"Don't blame my work on anything other than healing my body. *I interrupted the doctor.* Did you forget holistic healing was around way before medicine? You have no idea what I have experienced and what I have done. This hospital has done nothing for me other than make things worse. So, either you will order the MRI, test the worms or write my referral to see a parasitologist or this conversation is over."

"I've been very patient and listened to what you have said. But I don't think you have a parasite infection."

"You don't know what I have; you don't know what life was like for me last year when I suffered badly and thought I was going to die. You don't even know what it looks like to have a parasite infection. You studied medicine; I studied biology, microbiology, and parasitology. I am not trying to hear you tell me what's wrong, or what I should or shouldn't do. That's your problem; you have your belief system and are incapable of hearing anything else. You doctors think you know everything and you don't. So again, either you order an arthropod test, set up an MRI or write the script for the parasitologist."

"I can write the script for infectious disease. But do you want to see someone here or do you want to go to U I C?"

"I don't want to see anyone here."

"Okay, I will write the script."

177

Dr. Alexander stuck his hand out, and I shook it as I looked him square in his eyes. I wanted to punch him dead in his mouth.

Dr. Alex walked out the room, and I was pissed off. I was highly upset as these so-called doctors are either stupid or highly indoctrinated. But, I believe majority of them know parasites cause all disease. Why would he refuse to have the worms tested? I have good insurance. Why did he decline? Was he afraid of what the results would reveal? Was he afraid of a lawsuit?

You're probably wondering how that experience raised my vibrations. Well, after this past year of dealing with those doctors at the University of Chicago hospital, there was confirmation that no one is in charge of my health but me. It didn't make sense to go back to any appointments as I have done the work and continued to do so. I am my doctor and cannot be mad at someone who is clueless about parasites and yeast. Medical doctors know just enough to write a script and make an appointment. Other than that, they do not understand healing the body. But, still, I am grateful for the experience as it led me to take control of my health.

The following day, I stopped by Choice of Life, Holistic Wellness Center to set up an appointment for hydrotherapy. I also had dialogue with the practitioners. I chatted with one of the certified holistic health practitioners. I showed him the old images of my skin and the worms and he was amazed. In fact, he asked Dr. Robertson to take a look at the photos, and he was just as shocked. Both of them immediately identified the images as worms and candida yeast. This was the area that they specialized in as they have seen thousands of worms flush from colons as they perform hydrotherapy. I scheduled my appointment for November 4th. The day before my appointment, Dr. Mason from the University of Chicago hospital called me at home and offered to write a prescription for Nystatin (yeast) and Albendazole. I tried the nystatin as you gargle with it a few times a day, but I didn't feel comfortable killing the natural yeast in my mouth making room for other dis-ease. However, I did take the Albendazole.

Albendazole is used in the treatment of parasitic worm infestation such as giardiasis, trichuriasis, filariasis, pinworm, and neurocysticersis.

During my hydrotherapy appointment with Choice of Life on November 4th, 2017, I was told that some worms were still present and I believed them. During the procedure, I watched the tubing system as feces flowed through. The practitioner let me know when worms were passed. I also saw yeast. You have to understand that these little creatures lived in me for over 38 years and I knew it wouldn't be easy ridding my body of them and especially since there were 4 different worms. I believe the ones that were seen in the tubing were the round worms as they hang out in the skin area. I still felt them moving around, but the anal itch was long gone and so was the pain.

CHAPTER THIRTEEN

Pain Creates Power and Purpose

At 38 years young, I discovered that I came to this Earth school to not only heal the masses using my personal experiences, but to heal the lifetimes of pain my person has experienced. If you have read any of my books, you would know that I have experienced more pain than the average person and has worked my but off to heal and help you heal. The work I do is at the soul level. The work of healing has been more abundant that any amount of money I made during my "clock" days and now. I appreciate the "work" as it has led me to understand and appreciate shame, grief, guilt, apathy, anger, pride and desire, as well as willingness, acceptance, neutrality, love, peace, reason, joy and enlightenment. There is no light without darkness and there is no darkness without light. Pain is an experience suffering is the choice not to forgive and move through life angry and blaming. What purpose does anyone serve the world moving through angry and projecting pain onto others? Yes, there is pain in power, but how does one live in abundance and suffer at the same time. Pain is no stranger to abundance in some folk's lives as it wasn't a stranger to me. But I created it and as long as I am accountable, I can create something else, like, love, joy and peace that lead to wisdom.

Wisdom is nothing but healed pain as no one can teach it to you. Wisdom is the quality of having experience, knowledge, and good judgment. Experience is learned via lessons, not theoretically. There is a huge difference. Why is this important? Your experiences provide you with a lesson that only your experience can teach and provide wisdom. If 5 men experienced emotional trauma and tried to teach it to you, they would fail. The only way you gain wisdom and good judgement is via experience. I know what it feels like to burn from parasites toxins released into my bloodstream, as I also know how to heal.

That is wisdom; not everyone has it and not everyone has experienced it. But, one thing is for sure, everyone has experienced pain.

From the time I can remember, pain dominated my life and with each experience, I thought I was a victim. The more mentally and emotionally evolved I became the more I learned to appreciate the hand I was not only dealt, but created for myself. I was never a victim. My life was Perfectly Planned and always has been. It is unfortunate that we have all been trained to behave as victims and not creators. In order to heal, one has to be accountable for his or her presence and actions. Nothing happens to us unless we are in the space where it can occur and that alone makes us accountable. Accountability is very different from fault as you are responsible for you and everything in your life. What's more, we create everything we experience based on what we think and feel. You might find that hard to believe and continue to go through life blaming, but if you want health, wealth and success, you must create it. The only way that can happen is if you first heal and get the lesson so that you grow and don't repeat the experience. That was my life. A life of repeated experienced as I had no idea how to heal, be accountable, or look at self.

A term called introspection means to look at self. Most people are good at looking at self - in the mirror that is - but when it comes to looking deep within and looking at emotions, behaviors and thought process, the average person avoids it. Even after introspection, accountability and correction has to be applied or experiences repeat themselves. The fear is looking at your truth as that truth isn't always pretty. However, it is the ugly truth that creates beautiful people and pain that creates power and purpose. Every individual in this world that uses his or her life to help others has an ugly truth and capable of empowering others with that truth.

Introspection is important as it helps you to keep an eye on your development as a person. It also allows us to self-reflect and correct, assess your mental state, and understand your experience. Without introspection, there is not much spiritual growth, emotional intelligence or mental stability.

Another characteristic I developed via pain was vulnerability. My level of vulnerability is quite impressive and most people fear it. Vulnerability is the ability to be emotionally naked or physically exposed while risking attack and not concern oneself with what others think, say or feel. It is an enormous strength and people who suffer look for this characteristic in those who assist in healing. However, there are some who perceive vulnerability as weak as the European's man's definition is helpless, defenseless, powerless, impotent, weak, and susceptible. Vulnerability is far from any of those terms. It doesn't make me weak to say I have slept with over 100 men, or attempted suicide twice or released hundreds of worms from my body and nor does it make me helpless, powerless, or susceptible. It makes me strong, compassionate and empowered. What exactly am I susceptible to? Am I susceptible to an attack from someone? In the world we live in, people criticize those who share 'good' news so why would I care what someone thinks of me for sharing information that will help others? Vulnerability is extremely great place to be and without it, I would not be able to help you.

Transparency is another characteristic I allowed as I moved through my pain. Transparency is the ability to be seen clearly. I have no problem sharing my experiences to the world in an effort to heal and help you heal. It is what I do. Some people may not understand, however, my life isn't for others to understand, yet get some understanding of what healing is. I transparently transform lives worldwide and it is a blessing to do so. Transparency, like vulnerability is a sense of freedom as in not attempting to impress, be accepted by, or live by societal norms and conditioning. Without transparency, how can anyone see the truest and deepest parts of me? I know some people don't want to be seen as they haven't accepted themselves, so there is fear of criticism and rejection from others. I accept all of me and that is why it is easy for me to allow you to see all of me, like intimacy; (in to me I see).

My pain has allowed me to become a very empathetic person as I feel what isn't expressed, see what isn't shown and hear what isn't said. I care for people from a deep rooted place within me. I want people to heal and create happiness. More than often, I find myself intertwined in dark places or alone so that I can gain a better understanding of the world we live in. In the dark, there is light. Most of my clients have experienced great darkness and their information helps me to understand that until we all heal we will continue to project pain onto others as hurt people, hurt people. It is time for healed people to heal people.

As a healed person, a part of my ascension is the ability to be compassionate even to those people society considers the lowest; child molesters and rapist. People as such are suffering. If you squeeze a lemon what do you get? You get lemon juice. Well, if you come across a person who is emotionally and mentally suffering, what exactly do you think that person is going to give you? All they can give you is pain and misery. I am not making excuses rather pointing out the facts and they are, hurt people, hurt people. So with understanding that, I must have compassion for those people as well. Who will help them heal? Who will have understanding for their deep-rooted pain? In my pain, I hurt many, many people and I needed compassion. I needed someone to show me compassion. Compassion is a deep awareness of the suffering of someone along with the desire or wish to relieve it. I have compassion for even those who molest and rape.

I know that might be hard to believe for someone who has experienced sexual abuse and rape, but remember I know those things happened for me. Those experiences are the reason I am able to help transform lives worldwide. It was that pain that created power and purpose.

In essence, all of my experiences created the woman the world knows today. I would not be accountable, practice introspection, express vulnerability and transparency, or have a compassionate heart had I not experienced the tragedies that I did. Lastly, I am a wealth of knowledge and or wisdom. All that pain created power that led to purpose. I would not be interested in helping you had I not experienced what I have. Do you actually believe if I had not experienced sexual abuse, I would have two books on it? I would not deeply understand domestic violence had I not experienced it and took a good look at how I created that experience. I would not have six books, or be a professional speaker without my experiences. Those experiences were for my highest good, and for me to heal at the soul level and inspire you to be your best self.

I will always be in a space of growing and maturing. Personal development is required in order to reach your best self. When you stop learning, you stop living. Always be open to receive those who tell you the truth about you. Don't run from those people. In fact run to them and listen with an open mind. Relationships are required for spiritual growth. The only way a person can develop or grow by themselves is if they know how to self-reflect and correct. Without that ability, you will remain the same person and go through life complaining, only to find out later that you are your biggest challenge.

All of my challenges motivated me to self-reflect and correct or do what I call W.O.R.K; Willingly Open and Receive Knowledge. So many people resist knowledge as their mindsets are in a state of "I know." The moment you say I know, is the moment you missed the lesson. Always be willing to do the work. *Willingly open yourself* up to receive *knowledge* and always be grateful.

CHAPTER FOURTEEN

Gratitude

I asked for everything I received since August 2016. I created a vision board before my healing crisis and on it was a cigarette with an X marked through it. There were also images of vegan foods, green juices, an old picture of me weighing 135 pounds and so much more. The one thing I didn't request was how I wanted to manifest these things. I didn't plan as I merely asked. The Universe always says yes whether you wanted it or not, if you focus on it, be prepared to receive.

I got everything I asked for so how can I be mad. I wanted health and wellness, but to get that I had to heal first. To recover, I had to acknowledge the dis-ease. In doing so, my entire vision board came in full circle. It happened at a painful price, but it was well worth it. If the skin issue had never arrived, I would have never known about Mr. Parasite and Ms. Yeast. What's more, after learning about mucoid plaque and it's relation to constipation, polyps, and diverticulitis, my healing crisis could have very well been colon cancer. I cannot tell you how grateful I am for this experience. I feel like the yeast and parasites saved my life. I mean, knowing they were present in my body, is the reason I cleansed my colon and detoxed my organs. I wanted to be free of nicotine and alcohol and what better way to create transformation other than dis-ease. If dis-ease doesn't raise your vibrations, then I don't know what will.

I have nothing but gratitude for my healing crisis as you know I am a firm believer in pain is power and look at the power that has arisen out of Mr. Parasite and Ms. Yeast showing up. I am no longer a smoker; I don't drink alcohol, I released forty-five pounds of waste, I eat 95 percent clean and plant-based foods, my body is healthy and alive, I know how to heal my body as I have created optimal health. What more can I ask for? Life is good and better every day.

The education system teaches you and then tests you. Life examines you, and later you learn, that is if you choose to get the lesson. If we could become better Earth school students and focus on the teaching versus the experience, healing would be natural. It is unfortunate that we were all trained and programmed to blame and suffer. No one is responsible for my healing crisis as no one is responsible for my healing except me. I must continue to seek the lesson in every experience as I have suffered long enough. When you don't know how to heal whether it is emotional, mental, physical or soulful, you suffer. What's more, without gratitude there is no lesson, only continued suffering.

If I were to look back, I would not change one thing. All of that experience was FOR me, and now I can share it with you. I hope your heart fills with as much gratitude as mine is after you finish reading Detox or DIEt.

In fact, now that you are done, read it again and this time take notes as I am sure you will learn something different each time you read Detox or Diet. The following pages speak specifically to eliminating parasites from your body. But know this, you have to cleanse your colon and detox your elimination channels first. Worms and yeast will not leave your body if food is readily available to them. Give them a reason to leave. Clean house.

CHAPTER FIFTEEN

Natural Healing Remedies

Here you will find herbs and remedies that kill yeast and worms as well as heal the gut. Also, the article entitled *How to Get the Bugs Out* was written by Dr. Hull as she permitted me to use her article via email. Many of the herbs and supplements she wrote about are ones that I used and some I currently use today.

How To Get The Bugs Out
Dr. Janet Star Hull

Many diseases and disease syndromes source to parasites, bacteria, yeast or fungus. Here are some natural ways to prevent microorganisms from finding a home inside your body, and ways to remove them if they have already set up housekeeping. If microbes are present, certain foods, medications, and food chemicals can stimulate them. However, you may have unknowingly contracted microbes years ago, yet they have remained dormant. Ask yourself: did you ever cut your foot in a lake, or deal with animals? Where and when could you have picked them up?

Fungus or bacteria generally refer to Candida (yeast) and a variety of bacteria or fungi. Remember to avoid all sugars, food chemicals, and fermented foods if you suspect having microbes. Fermentation feeds microorganisms. A colon cleanse is recommended when detoxing from microbes to help secure their healthy removal - all the way out of your body. At the first sign of health symptoms returning, begin another round of cleansing supplements until symptoms completely disappear.

If you suspect having parasites within you may be contributing to the root of your health concerns and to the root of many cancers, more specific nutrients may be necessary to remove them. Interestingly, I have discovered through years of performing the hair analyses that parasites (including most bacteria) attach to toxic metals (such as lead, mercury, copper or titanium) like barnacles attach to a ship! It is important to remove them all.

PARASITE DESTROYERS

BLACK WALNUT - The dried and ground green hull of the Black Walnut contains tannin, which is organic iodine, as well as juglandin, extractive matter from the juice of the green shucks of the walnut. Black walnut has been used for centuries to expel various types of worms, including parasites that cause skin irritations such as ringworm. It oxygenates the blood, which also helps kill parasites. Black Walnut is very effective against tapeworms, pinworms, Candida albicans (yeast infections) and malaria. It is also effective in reducing blood sugar levels, and helping the body rid itself of toxins.

WORMWOOD - This is one of the MOST POWERFUL tools in the parasite-killing herb kingdom. It is most effective against roundworms, hookworms, whipworms and pinworms. Wormwood contains the potent chemicals thujone and isothujone, which are the primary components that kill parasites. Wormwood also contains santonin, an effective remedy for parasitic diseases.

Wormwood is the second most bitter herb known to man and has been proven as a POWERFUL remedy for malaria. Wormwood also contains sesquiterpene lactones, which work similarly to peroxide by weakening the parasites membranes therefore killing them. Wormwood also helps produce bile, which in turn helps the liver and gallbladder.

CLOVES - Cloves contain eugenol, caryophyllene, and tannins, which are powerful antimicrobial agents. These components travel through the bloodstream, killing microscopic parasites and parasitic larvae and eggs. Eugenol has a pleasant, spicy, clove-like odor, and is the main biologically active compound in clove cigarettes. Cloves are tremendously effective in killing malaria, tuberculosis, cholera, scabies and other parasites, viruses, bacteria and fungi, including Candida. Cloves also destroy Pseudomonas aeruginosa (a pathogen from plants), all species of Shigella, Staphylococcus, and Streptococcus.

THYME - Thyme contains flavonoids that are most commonly known for their antioxidant activity, and thymol and carvacrol, which are effective in killing bacteria, fungal infections, and yeast infections. Thyme is especially effective in killing hook-worms, roundworms, threadworms and skin parasites. Thyme also destroys Cryptococcus neoformans, Aspergillus, Saprolegnia, Salmonella typhimurium, Staphylococcus aureas, and Escherichia coli.

Used as an antibiotic, thymol is 25 times more effective than phenol (a manufactured substance found in a number of consumer products known to cause liver damage), yet less toxic to parasites. Thyme is the primary ingredient in the original LISTERINE® MOUTHWASH because of its germ killing power.

HYSSOP - Hyssop contains essential hormone oil that is very effective in destroying a variety of parasites and is very effective against the herpes simplex virus.

GARLIC - Garlic is known to slow and kill more than 60 types of fungi and 20 types of bacteria, as well as some of the most potent viruses known to humans. Garlic has a history of killing parasites and controlling secondary fungal infections, detoxifying while gently stimulating elimination, and has antioxidant properties to protect against oxidation caused by parasite toxins.

Allicin and Ajoene are the components in garlic that kill parasites, including one-cell varieties, as well as pinworms and hookworms. Allicin is not present in garlic in its natural state. When garlic is chopped or otherwise damaged, the enzyme alliinase acts on the chemical alliin converting it into allicin. Ajoene is the principal chemical responsible for garlic's anticoagulant properties and contributes to its strong odor.

189

Garlic has antimicrobial properties, including antibacterial, antiviral, antifungal, antiprotozoal, and antiparasitic, that kills: B. subtilis, E. coli, P. mirabilis, Salmonella typhi, Salmonella enteritidis, methicillin-resistant Staph aureus, Staph faecalis, and V. cholerae, Staphylococcus, Escherichia, Proteus, Salmonella, Providencia, Citrobacter, Klebsiella, Hafnia, Aeromonas, Vibrio and Bacillus genera. Garlic is also very effective against Mycobacterium tuberculosis. Garlic has also been known to eliminate Candida albicans.

FENNEL - This herb is known to be antiparasitic. Fennel seed is used to help remove and expel parasites and their wastes. Fennel is also very effective against Candida albicans.

CAYENNE - A member of the Capsicum genus, known for assisting with assimilation, healing, improved circulation, cleansing, indigestion, urinary tract health, colds, flu and other benefits too numerous to mention, cayenne also destroys parasites.

GINGER - The components of gingerol, the active constituent of fresh ginger, destroys parasites including the roundworm, the blood fluke, the anisakid worm, and the Salmonella bacteria.

GENTIAN - This herb is wonderful for ridding the body of parasites including plasmodia, which is a malaria-causing parasite. Gentian is also good for treating anemia and counteracting the effects of parasite toxins in the body by stimulating the liver to produce more bile.

BODY & BLOOD PURIFIERS THAT REMOVE TOXINS

MILK THISTLE - Silymarin is the primary component in Milk Thistle that removes liver toxins. Milk Thistle promotes liver cell regeneration, and its antioxidant action protects against cell damage from toxins. Milk Thistle is most helpful in cleansing the toxins given off by parasites.

MARSHMALLOW ROOT - Marshmallow Root contains mucilage, a gummy substance obtained from certain plants. When Marshmallow Root gets wet, it becomes soft and sticky, which soothes the mouth, throat, stomach and intestinal tract. When parasites are dislodged from body tissue, they can leave an open sore. Marshmallow Root coats these sores so there is less irritation.

PAU D' ARCO- Pau d'Arco is used for Candida, yeast infections, fungal infections, viral infections, and parasitic infections. It also helps relieve cystitis, prostatitis, ringworm, gonorrhea, and syphilis. Pau d'Arco is one of the most powerful antioxidants known, and stimulates the immune system. Pau d'Arco also helps relieve leaky bladder syndrome.

BURDOCK - Burdock removes accumulated waste and toxins from the skin, kidneys, mucous and serous membranes. A very effective blood purifier, Burdock is wonderful for head, face and neck skin problems including, Eczema , Psoriasis, boils, carbuncles, eyesores, and dermatitis.

ELECAMPANE - This herb is to the lungs what Marshmallow Root is to the digestive tract. It is a natural expectorant, which helps coat and soothe the lungs as impurities are coughed up and expelled. Elecampane also has an antibacterial effect that purifies the lungs.

FENUGREEK - This herb works very much like elecampane with an added blood purifying quality.

LICORICE - Licorice is also an expectorant and demulcent just like elecampane and fenugreek. It also is an anti-inflammatory, anti-spasmodic and mild laxative. It purifies the organs and the endocrine system, especially the liver.

COLON & BOWEL HELPERS
BARBERRY - The ingredients of Barberry, columbamine, berberine, and oxyacanthine, have antibacterial and antiviral

properties. *Research indicates that berberine in Barberry is specifically effective against cholera, giardia, Shigella, Salmonella and E. coli. The berberines aid in the secretion of bile and are good for liver problems. Barberry is also a mild laxative, and helps the digestive processes. Barberry also helps with Staphylococcus, Streptococcus, Salmonella, cholera and chronic candidiasis (yeast). Berberines are highly bactericidal, amoeboidal and trypanocidal.*

Barberry acts the same as chloramphenicol, a commonly prescribed antibiotic drug. Barberry helps to purify the respiratory and digestive systems, and also has an antiparasitic effect.

CASCARA SAGRADA - Also known as Buckthorn, Cascara Sagrada stimulates increased wavelike contractions of the large intestines. Cascara has also been known to expel parasites through its wavelike actions in the lower intestines, and is highly recommended during parasite removal. Cascara Sagrada is considered one of the safest laxatives, and is useful in detoxifying the colon.

SENNA - Senna is a powerful laxative that is excellent for expelling worms. Senna works best when combined with other anthelmintic herbs (used in the treatment of roundworm), such as ginger or fennel. These herbs increase regularity and reduce the chance of bowel cramps due to Senna's strong action. Senna effectively cleans the elimination system, and has a vermifuge action that repels parasites. Senna is the ingredient in many over-the-counter laxatives, including Fletcher's Castoria[a], Senokot[a] and Innerclean Herbal Laxative.

SAGE - Sage has the power to relax the muscles lining the digestive tract. Sage contains relatively high levels of thujone which is the same ingredient in wormwood that kills parasites. Sage is also used to increase circulation, and is considered an excellent remedy for poor digestion and stomach problems.

PSYLLIUM - Removes toxins from the colon and is especially useful in cleaning out all of the pockets in the colon wall. Psyllium swells up to 50 times its size, and is powerfully effective in removing waste and toxins from the colon.

YELLOW DOCK - Works as a laxative, but unlike other laxatives, yellow dock also promotes bile flow, which purifies the blood. It is rich in digestible iron that helps restore blood nutrients to the body.

CRAMP BARK - The components of Cramp Bark (Vitamin K, viburnin, isovalerianic acid, hydroquinines, coumarins, salicin, salicosides, arbutin, sterol, tannin, and resin) greatly calm gastrointestinal cramping by relaxing the smooth muscles. It also helps with general muscle cramping; reducing any cramping that might occur while the colon is working to expel parasites.

PEPPERMINT - Peppermint is well known for relieving indigestion, but it also relaxes the stomach muscles, relieves gas, and is also good for nausea and vomiting. Peppermint also has antiparasitic properties.

End Article

CHAPTER SIXTEEN

Conclusion

In conclusion, allopathy treatment served its purpose of creating billions of dollars for the elite as healing dis-ease was never the end-goal. The sole focus was to generate income, build capitalism and a medical monopoly. Why not combine the two, medicine and holistic healing, instead of burying holistic healing and making the entire industry illegal unless one has a medical doctoral degree. How does bleeding people, removing body parts and prescribing drugs support our health? It does not and never will. Rockefeller practically owns the world, and if you think for one minute he is concerned about your health and wellness, you are sadly mistaken. Medicine is money and has never surrounded healing. Sure, doctors prescribe a pill to cure dis-ease, and sometimes that pill or chemical works, but that same pill or chemical kills your natural bacteria, creates a toxic and acidic environment and causes more dis-ease to fester. What's more, steroids are known to compromise the immune system. Healing means to restore the body's natural ability to fight off dis-ease as it does not say to suppress the body's immune system while affording pathogens the means to resist drugs and take over our bodies. In my eyes, the healthcare industry is no different than any other sector as it is all about the bottom line, money, and unfortunately, at the expense of our health and wellness and that includes mental and emotional health.

Please do not underestimate the power of your emotions as they are at the center of which you are as without them, you may as well consider yourself a robot. In order to heal, we have to feel. When you avoid or suppress your emotions, you also ignore the manifestation of physical dis-ease. The willingness to look at the emotional aspect of physical pain or injury leads to releasing emotional toxins resulting in healing. There is no physical dis-ease without first, emotional dis-ease. Mind-body disorders are real and it doesn't matter if the pain stems from a physical injury, there are unhealthy emotions attached first. We have been so

194

deeply programmed to avoid, turn a blind eye to and ignore our deepest feelings using materials, relationships and money that we have no idea we create dis-ease. Everything starts in your head. If you have stinking thinking, toxic emotions follow. We have to give ourselves permission to feel and release sadness, anger, guilt or embarrassment; acknowledge the presence of it and then release it via tears. Those tears carry toxins just as sweat does. Release them and stop behaving like a robot. Acknowledge the pain and agony that exist in your mind. Don't pretend like all is well and then when you get sick; you behave like a victim. Look within and identify why you feel miserable and if you need assistance moving through your emotions, you are welcome to reach out to me. Trust me, you do not want to experience what I have, and if you have, that burning from the inside is enough to make anyone cry.

Today, I understand that burning was directly related to my toxic gut and the inability to release toxins due to my blocked colon. I also understand the role played by the intestinal worms, candida yeast, GMO's, alcohol and my toxic emotions. The best part about this experience was that I learned how to heal my body. I know for sure that all dis-ease starts in the gut and if I feel any burning, spiking or any symptom, you better believe I'm scheduling an appointment for hydrotherapy and detoxification. I will not run to conventional doctors as I know now that they are clueless or deeply brainwashed and will only misdiagnose me.

My self-diagnosis was on point and without the use of the internet, 23 years in healthcare, medical books and research, I highly doubt if I would have figured out the Leaky Gut. It's one thing to have intestinal parasites and an overgrowth of yeast, but it's another situation when the yeast and worms leave the intestine and make their way into your skin. Leaky Gut is more common in the world than most people know or doctors are even interested in. I've been told by several conventional doctors that you cannot test for Leaky Gut and that no test exists. I beg to differ. I have talked to several naturopath doctors who examine for Leaky Gut and treat it with supplements. Although the self-diagnosis was correct, it still doesn't rule out the fact that the overgrowth of yeast and intestinal parasites were present in my body. The diagnosis that was absurd was the Lichen Planus.

Conventional medicine has everyone thinking that Psoriasis, Lichen Planus, Eczema and Pityriasis Rosacea are skin disorders and that there are no cures. Skin disorders are symptoms of a toxic gut, and it doesn't matter what's toxins are present, your colon needs flushing so that the small bowels can release. Skin disorders are merely symptoms of a septic tank. The only solution is to cleanse your colon and stop ingesting toxins. And don't even bother with light therapy and steroids.

I had a few people tell me light therapy worked for them and others said it didn't work. Well, the few treatments I had was a waste of my time. Treating symptoms is not the preferred method. You have to address the cause and that is a toxic gut. Light therapy is no different than a tanning booth, as mentioned, on one occasion my skin blistered, and that was my last time going. For those who were successfully treated by the light therapy, be aware as the symptoms will come back until you detox your body and flush your colon. Worms and yeast love waste, but they hate turpentine.

The turpentine and castor oil worked well, however, even with that protocol, I wasn't finished cleansing my body. The amount of mucus I released was unreal. Mucus is a breeding ground for bacteria, intestinal worms, yeast or any other pathogen. And an overproduction of mucus signifies many disorders and a parasitic infection is one of them. After less than a week of taking the turpentine, I released hundreds of pinworms and lots of yeast. However, the majority of the worms were released after the mucoid plaque. The colon has to be cleaned before turpentine and castor oil can be one hundred percent effective. At any rate, I keep turpentine and castor oil in my supplement cabinet.

The detox and colon cleanse was the absolute best process ever. I released a total of twenty-five pounds of waste during this process and twenty before. It was also very challenging. However, I made it through feeling great, happy, healthy and ready to take on the world. I healed my thyroid, normalized my blood pressure, and lipid panels as I no longer have early-stage heart disease. There is only one cure or the human body, and that is to do seasonal detoxes and monthly hydrotherapy. What's more, preventative measures include eating organic, avoiding meat, processed foods and GMO's, and stop drinking alcohol and using drugs. As Americans, it is challenging to avoid toxins as this entire corporation (country) is toxic. The only way we can eliminate toxins is to leave this country and go somewhere where human life is appreciated and loved more than money.

The month of August was simultaneously surprising and traumatizing. Once I cleaned my colon, the long worms had no choice but to come out of me. Almost the entire month of August, I released worm after worm and several times my stool smelled of sewage. I do not have that problem today. This healing crisis has been the most influential experience I have ever endured. I understand that when abnormal symptoms appear, the body needs healing and if you respond immediately and detox and cleanse your colon, you can instantly stop the symptoms and heal your body. If I knew better at the beginning of my crisis, I would have immediately detoxed my body. No need to cry over spilled milk. The best part about this crisis is that my story touched the world. Today, I eat to live, although my eating habits aren't perfect, I am 85% better than what I was before this crisis. I intentionally seek organic foods and avoid GMO's. Now, when it comes to eating out, you just have no idea what you are eating so going out to dinner has decreased, unless the food is organic like True Kitchen in downtown Chicago. For the most part, I eat with the intention to live and not die. This illness has undoubtedly raised my vibrations as I took control of my health and healed my body. I researched daily, worked with naturopaths, plant practitioners, and a few others to gain the knowledge that I did. I am a healer, and no one can take that from me. My level of gratitude is at an all-time high as I realized my story is much bigger than me. People all across the world viewed my video as they needed to see someone who not only understood the pain but that the truth was within our colons and healing is possible. I would not change anything about this experience other than to do better from here on out.

2014-2016
Hypothyroidism, high cholesterol, high blood pressure and
early stage heart disease, 178 pounds

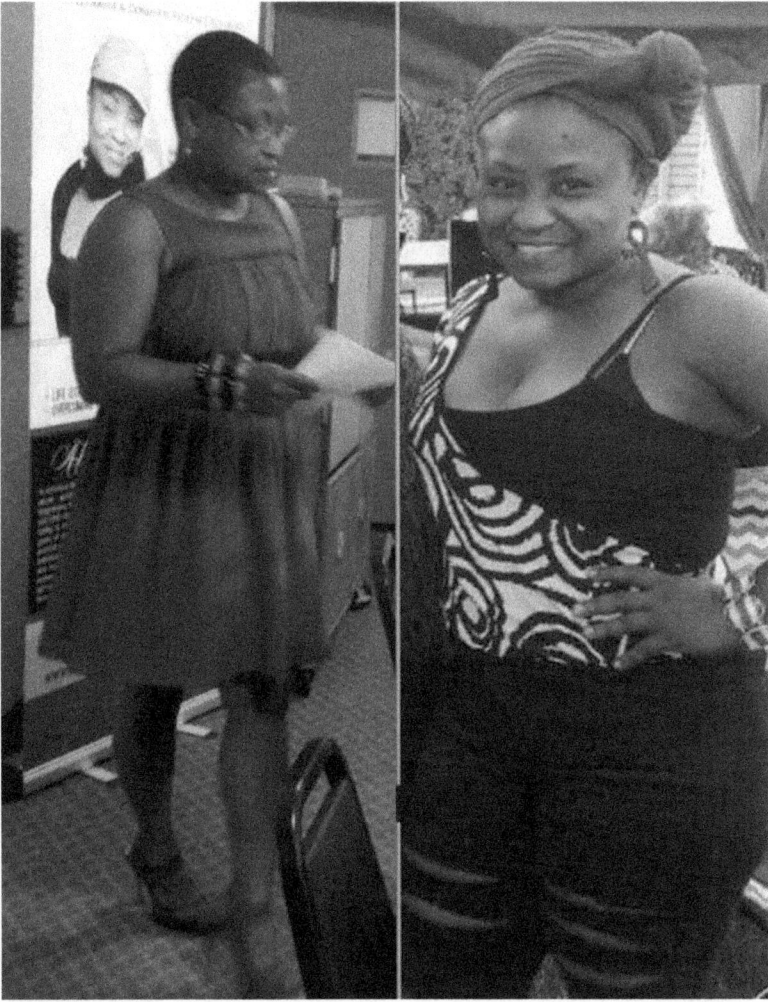

Today
Optimal Health: thyroid healed, normal blood pressure,
normal cholesterol, healthy heart, 133 pounds

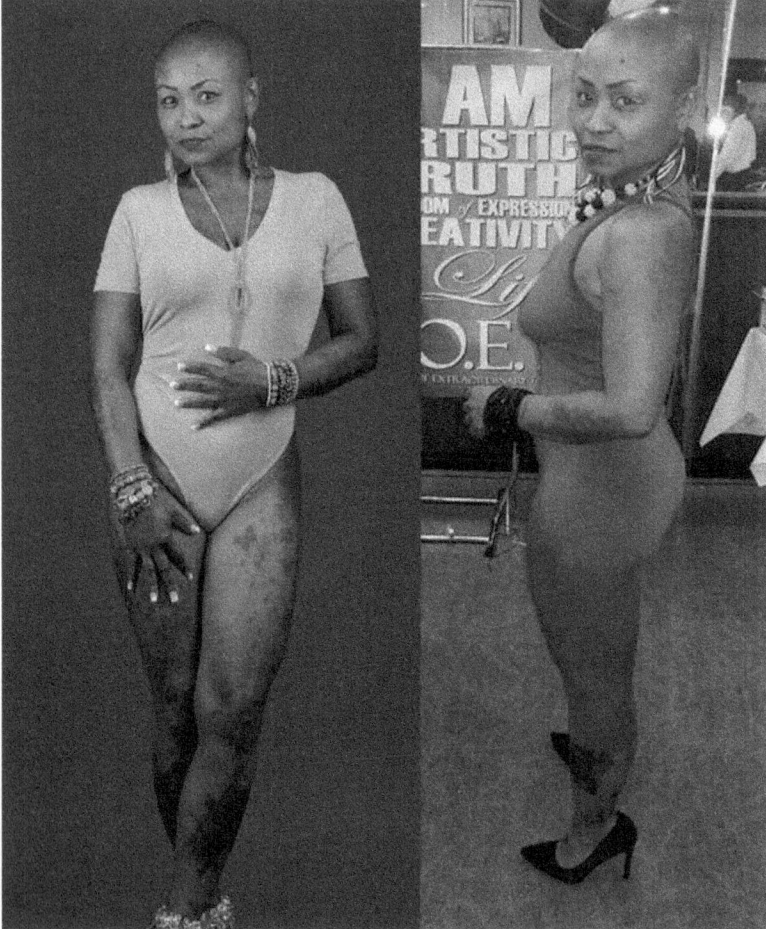

Epilogue

Today, I am doing very well. I currently take Dr. Axe's Candida Combat and well as intestinal repair or Leaky Gut repair. I have finally eliminated all the worms from my body and the yeast is balanced. I took my body back. I do not eat pork, beef, fish, or turkey, but I have not completely given up chicken. I might have it once or twice a week. For the most part, I am 95% vegetarian.

I didn't choose vegan as the vegan lifestyle feeds the yeast. There is too much consumption of beans, nuts and bread. Beans, nuts and bread feeds yeast as beans and nuts are molds and bread is yeast. I eat the garbanzo beans regularly. Vegans also consume a lot of fruits and sweet treats and although the sugar is a healthy sugar, it still feeds yeast. I am intentional about feeding my body and not my cohabitants.

Today I recommend a few things to maintain optimal health.
- Warm or hot lemon water for breakfast (24oz)
- Fast 4 hours upon rising
- Seasonal detoxes
- Monthly hydrotherapy
- Weekly enemas
- Monthly coffee enemas
- Daily probiotic (25-100 billion)
- Plant based diet
- Avoid all white foods and especially white bread
- Organic foods
- Clean your fruits and vegetables
- Take an Enzyme Digest
- Exercise 4 days a week (run, walk, jog)
- Drink half your body weight of water in ounces
- Avoid white sugar and sugary products

- Prop your feet up on a stool when pooping

Meat eaters
- Everything above along with the bullets below
- Bi-weekly hydrotherapy
- Bi-weekly enemas
- Bi-weekly coffee enemas
- Eat meat once a day, NOT all day
- Eat meat 3 times a week, NOT everyday
- Eat at least one good leafy salad daily

Be intentional about your health. This journey has taken me over a year to get to this space, so don't expect any overnight results. If it took you years to get to where you are, give yourself at least a year or more to recover and create optimal health. Do not go back to doing what you did before.

I hope Detox or DIEt has empowered, enlightened and transformed your life. The journey is never ending.

Have you ever traveled outside of America? i.e. China, Africa, Mexico or Europe?

Do you drink tap water?

Do you regular eat unpeeled raw fruits and raw vegetables?

Do you prefer meat, fish or poultry that is rare or medium rare?

Do you eat pork or any products containing pork?

Do you use the same cutting board for chicken, pork and meat as you do for your vegetables?

Do you eat raw dishes like sushi?

Do you have a dog?

Do you forget to wash your hands after petting your dog?

Does your pet eat from your plates?

Does your pet sleep in your bed?

Do you engage in oral sex?

Do you practice anal sex without condoms?

Are there dark circles under your eyes?

Do have allergies?

Do you have insomnia or wake up in the middle of the night between 2am and 3am?

Do you have persistent acne, Eczema, Psoriasis, Pityriasis Rosea, Lichen Planus or any other skin eruptions?

Do you have belly fat?

Do you experience anal itching?

Do you feel fatigued?

Do you experience creepy crawling, like something is crawling on your skin?

Do you have cravings?

Do you have digestive issues, i.e., Irritable Bowel Syndrome, intermittent diarrhea or constipation?

Do you have brain fog, i.e, forgetfulness, loss of words in the middle of a sentence?

If you answered yes to any of those questions, more than likely, you have parasites in your body. This is in no way a diagnosis rather an observation based on my direct experience.

The symptoms listed above can be due to other medical reasons; however, do not rule out the possibilities of parasites.

About the Author

A successful leader and expert on overcoming all forms of abuse, avoiding toxic relationships and the art of forgiveness, Kelley Porter is a Certified Transformation, and Personal Development Coach, Award Winning Six-time Author, and Professional Speaker. As a speaker, Kelley's transparent and authentic style of speaking will empower anyone to self-reflect, start the process of healing and correct thoughts and behaviors that may hinder them from living a healthy and non-toxic lifestyle.

As a Coach, Kelley empowers you to reach emotional freedom, gain clarity and discover your infinite possibilities. She is well known for assisting in the removal of mental and emotional blocks that hinders people from reaching their fullest potential. Her areas of specialty are, but not limited to; abuse, healing, relationships, thoughts, emotions, and behaviors as she has written books on all topics. Kelley has over thirty years of direct experience with all forms of abuse, domestic violence relationships, creating purpose and power from painful experiences, and creating a positive mindset.

Kelley contributes to society her genuine love for healing, improving awareness and identity, developing talents and potential; enhancing the quality of life and the realization of dreams and aspirations. Kelley's mission is to guide you to design a healthy and meaningful life through wisdom, consciousness, self-reflection, self-love, accountability and forgiveness. Prior to Kelley discovering her life purpose, she spent twenty-three years in healthcare and worked fifteen of those years as a Medical Technologist, as she is a member of the American Society for Clinical Pathologist.

Kelley has been seen and heard on radio and TV including WVON, HOT105 (Florida), Inspiration 1390, WKKC, Channel 2, 5, 7 and 19 and My Black is Beautiful (online). She has been featured in Rolling Out Magazine, Chicago Tribune, Bean Soup Times, SisterSpeak237 (Africa) and spoken for numerous prestigious organizations such as Robert H. McKinney Law School and the Chicago Police Department. She is available for speaking engagements such as keynotes, seminars, workshops, conferences and panels. Her audience can range from congregations, universities, youth groups, NFP and community organizations, the educational and prison system as well as shelters.

References

Amelong, K. (2017). Optimal Health Network: Therapeutic Grade Essential Oil Suppository Recipes. Retrieved from: http://www.optimalhealthnetwork.com/Therapeutic-Grade Essential-Oil-Suppository-Recipes-s/1195.htm

Anderson, R. (2017). Cleansing the Colon: The Key to Excellent Health Retrieved from: https://cdn.shopify.com/s/files/1/0783/4779/files/PC_COLON_ CLEANSE_Richard_Anderson_method.pdf

Aston, D. (2015). 10 Signs That You May Have A Parasite & How To Get Rid Of It! Retrieved from: http://www.whyamiunhealthy.com/contact-us/

Daniels, J. (1999). Confidential Underground Report: The Candida Cleaner. Retrieved from: http://candidacleaner.s3.amazonaws.com/The_Candida_Clea ner.pdf

Hull, J. (2011). How to Get the Bugs Out. Parasite Destroyers http://www.janethull.com/newsletter/0107/how_to_get_the_bu gs_out_1.php

Kulkarni, T. (2016). 8 Things That Happen When You Don't Sweat Retrieved from: https://www.boldsky.com/health/wellness/2016/eight-things-that-happen-when-you-dont-sweat-100111.html

Last, W. (Year unknown). Turpentine Therapy: Rectified Oil of Turpentine, Rectified Turpentine Oil. Retrieved from http://augmentinforce.50webs.com/TURPENTINE--HEALER%20COMPLETE.htm#TURPENTINE--HEALER COMPLETE

Maeda, K. (2016) Gut Microbiome. Retrieved from
   http://katmaeda.com/why-did-hippocrates-say-all-disease-
   begins-in-the-gut/

Stagg, J. (2016). HOW TOXIC THOUGHTS DESTROY YOUR
   HEALTH: THE DNA CONNECTION. Retrieved from
   http://www.drstagg.com/toxic-thoughts-destroy-health-dna-
   connection/

Stoppler, C. (2003). M.Melanosis Coli (Pseudomelanosis Coli)
   Retrieved from
   https://www.medicinenet.com/melanosis_coli/article.htm#what
   _is_melanosis_coli

Zoldan, J. (year unknown). Candida Syndrome. Retrieved from
   http://www.drjackzoldan.com/Candida-Syndrome.html
Unknown Year and /or Unlisted Authors

Chemometec. (2017). Retrieved from
   https://chemometec.com/applications/somatic-cell-counting/

Cleaning Up the Mess After the Floor or Sewage Back-Up. (Year
   unknown). Retrieved from
   https://genoa.org/articles/article/sewerbackupcleanup

Guest Contributor. (2015). 15 Health Problems Linked to
   Monsanto's Roundup. Retrieved from
   https://www.ecowatch.com/15-health-problems-linked-to-
   monsantos-roundup-1882002128.html

Mayo Clinic Staff. (2017). Trans fat is double trouble for your
   heart Retrieved from https://www.mayoclinic.org/diseases-
   conditions/high-blood-cholesterol/in-depth/trans-fat/art-
   20046114

Perfect Health "The Candida Diet" (Year unknown). Retrieved
   from https://www.thecandidadiet.com/candida-die-off-
   symptoms/

Nature Remedies: The Natural Choice. (Year unknown). Retrieved fromhttp://www.nativeremedies.com/ingredients/reduce-disruptive-behavior-with-hyoscyamus.html

Probacto: Candida Die-Off: (2013). Everything You Need to Know About Herxheimer Candida Die Off. Retrieved from http://blog.probacto.com/everything-you-need-to-know-about-herxheimer-candida-die-off/

www.ingramcontent.com/pod-product-compliance
Lightning Source LLC
Chambersburg PA
CBHW032134020426
42334CB00016B/1165